Had we a
behind the bible, we would all
have been enslaved by the
Nazi's and the barbaric,
imperial, tyrants.

:60 Second
Chronic Pain Relief

:60 Second Chronic Pain Relief

The Quickest Way to Soften the Throb, Cool the Burn, Ease the Ache

by Peter G. Lehndorff, M.D.
with Brian Tarcy

NEW HORIZON PRESS
Far Hills, New Jersey

Requests for permission should be addressed to:
New Horizon Press
P.O. Box 669
Far Hills, NJ 07931

Lehndorff, Peter G. with Tarcy, Brian.
        :60 Second Chronic Pain Relief
        The Quickest Way to Soften the Throb, Cool the
        Burn, Ease the Ache

Library of Congress Catalog Card Number: Pending

ISBN: 0-88282-151-2

New Horizon Press

Manufactured in the U.S.A.

2000 1999 1998 1997 / 5 4 3 2 1

Authors' Note

The material in this book is intended to provide a quick review of methods and information now available and to raise awareness to natural alternatives. Any of the treatments described herein for the alleviation of chronic pain symptoms should be discussed with a licensed health care practitioner. The authors and publisher assume no responsibility for any adverse outcomes which derive from use of any of these treatments in a program of self-care or under the care of a licensed practitioner.

The information in this book is based on Dr. Lehndorff's research and medical records of patients. Some names and identifying characteristics have been changed to protect the privacy of individuals.

Contents

Introduction

Every individual is unique and experiences pain differently. You may ask, what is this book going to tell me about chronic pain? Well, the first thing is that no one strategy works for everyone. You may think, after years of pain, that you have tried everything to cure it and the only answer is to endure suffering.

But you are wrong.

No matter what knowledge you have accumulated, if you still are pain ridden, you can do better.

No one strategy works, but there is a *philosophy* that is essential. A philosophy of curiosity and courage, one that says you can change your life.

Chronic pain. Even the words hurt. It is a condition that hardly ever goes away. It is like repetitive bad music, but hurting the body as well as the soul. It can ruin your life if you let it.

I have seen many battles with chronic pain. In my

1

long medical career, I have seen thousands of patients fighting pain.

Not long ago, I realized I had a wealth of information about pain. In order to discover some remedies which really work, I decided to survey the thousands of patients' records I had accumulated.

My name is Dr. Peter G. Lehndorff. I began my career as an anesthesiologist and then developed a speciality in pain control. After that, I headed a pain clinic. I am going to write this book as if you were visiting my office and needed help. I have been dedicated to the relief of pain all my life. Let me share with you what I have learned.

I have seen chronic pain so bad that even the name of the sufferer's disease hurt. Just thinking about it hurts. Aches. Throbs. Pains. I've witnessed them all, in different areas of the body. In addition, as a person growing older, I've felt chronic pain myself.

In my long career, I have formulated theories about the best way to manage pain. One of the things that I have noticed is that there is a difference between those who improved and those who did not. This was true whatever the type or degree of pain suffered. Some patients didn't improve, though virtually every treatment method was tried. Some just got better naturally while others didn't.

On the other hand, a good number of other patients improved greatly and sooner than expected. I focused on this successful group, for I believed they could provide clues as to how to improve treatment for those who don't get well.

First I looked at treatments, many of which we shall discuss, including: vitamin therapy, special exercises, nerve blocks, electric stimulators, ointments, medications, hypnosis, and counseling. Some worked for particular patients and didn't work for others. However, no one treatment worked every time.

I began to look further, wanting to discern a pattern of success. I found none until I looked at attitude. The patients who showed the most and fastest improvement shared only one characteristic: the urgent desire and will to improve.

The mind has immense powers. We can do the most surprising things if we are properly motivated. There are proven methods to stimulate motivation. Other treatments also need to be considered. I will discuss many in these pages, but you must understand that they don't always work, and I think I know why. In fact, I am sure I know why.

Attitude. Yes. Optimism or pessimism.

•The patients who succeeded *wanted* to get better.
•They *expected* to get better.
•They *worked* on getting better.
•They *learned* quick methods of motivation.

I truly believe motivation is a key to conquering chronic pain. So, first I offer many tools to learn :60 second attitude adjustments.

Chapter 1

:60 SECONDS OF
INFORMATION
ABOUT PAIN

Something is wrong. You know that and I know that. That's why you've come to me. You have a throb, a burn, a pang, or an ache which recurs too frequently or is with you constantly. You have come to a pain specialist looking for answers.

Good for you.

You see, I am thrilled that you would choose to keep looking. No matter how long you have fought your chronic pain, I know that curiosity is the first step toward finding a cure. Wait. I am not talking about a cure for the physical cause of your pain (your doctor must treat this condition), but about learning to live with pain and making life better. This means not ignoring the pain, but rather attacking it.

:60 Second Plan of Attack

1.	First and foremost, attack the pain where you can do the most good—in your mind.
2.	Treatment and exercise.
3.	Understand your pain before attempting to alleviate it.

:60 Second Pain Definition

The official definition of *pain* as worked out by the International Association for the Study of Pain in Seattle is: an unpleasant sensory and emotional experience associated with actual or potential tissue damage, or described in terms of such damage.

There are two kinds of pain:

1. *Acute pain* is of a recent onset and probably limited duration. The pain usually starts near the area of the body that has undergone some trauma.

2. *Chronic pain* lasts for long periods of time. Chronic pain usually persists beyond the time of healing of an injury, and, frequently, there may not be any clearly identifiable cause.

Why is this? It is because pain is transmitted from the nerves, along the spine, and to the brain. When there is a damaged tissue from a cut, bruise, fracture, or an inflammation, certain signals are transmitted by nerve fibers. Depending on the nerve fiber, the pain felt will have specific characteristics. It may burn or throb, be sharp or dull.

The nerve fibers sole purpose is to relay signals to the brain. These signals differ depending on the situation as well as the location of the nerve.

Signals from the nerves are then transmitted via the spinal cord to the brain. In the spine, pain is modulated naturally. Pain can be weakened or reinforced in the spinal cord. If we did not have this mechanism we would always be in pain, even those who do not suffer from chronic pain. Everything that happens to us would hurt. Thankfully, our body fights back.

The Body Fights Back

The spine consists of a long line of bones called the vertebrae. These bones support the spine, and in between these bones there are joints which make the movement of your back and body possible.

Inside this column of vertebrae runs the spinal cord, consisting mainly of nerve cells and nerve fibers. These cells give life to nerve fibers, and direct the flow of signals through the fibers. These cells can either reinforce or weaken the signal considerably. In general, the posterior, or back, part of the spinal cord registers sensation and feeling. The anterior, or front, part of the cord specializes in motion.

The spinal cord reaches from the brain to the lower part of the back. If you were to cut your spinal cord across at any level, you would find that the outer part is whitish, and the center part is gray. The gray part has the shape of a butterfly, and the back part of the wing is called the posterior horn.

Many types of nerve fibers that transmit pain go into the posterior horn part of the spinal cord. Pain is processed in the posterior horn. Electrical and chemical signals come down from the centers in the brain, and can encourage the posterior horn to fight the pain.

There are two theories about how this works.

:60 Second Theories

1.   The first is the *Gate Theory*: Two different types of nerve fibers (thick and thin) meet in the posterior horn. The thick fibers conduct feelings and help us locate parts of our body. The thick fibers are stronger and faster than the thin ones that conduct pain.

When these two pain signals meet, the stronger signal tends to suppress the weaker. The doctors who worked on this theory (Dr. Ronald Melzack, Professor of Psychology at McGill University in Montreal, and Dr. Patrick D. Wall, Professor of Physiology at United Medical and Dental Schools in London) received a Nobel Prize for their work.

2.   The second theory is that the body produces chemicals called *endorphins* to help the body fight pain naturally. Endorphins function similarly to narcotics in their ability to block out pain. These

chemicals split off from the body's DNA.

DNA is the substance that controls the life of a cell and gives the cell orders to grow or stop growing. On the surface of cells, especially nerve cells, there are areas that receive narcotics or endorphins. One area where the body fights pain is in the opioid receptors.

When endorphins split off from DNA, they make life in normal circumstances painless by going into the opioid receptors. Although a detailed explanation of DNA would take several chapters, the important thing for a chronic pain sufferer to note is that the endorphins that come from DNA are natural substances you want to encourage.

Without endorphins, many normal events would be quite painful. This is noticeable in someone who has taken narcotics for a period of time. Narcotics have a tendency to saturate opioid receptors which can shut down the production of endorphins.

When there are no endorphins available, and if the intake of narcotics has stopped, the body goes through a painful process called withdrawal. In other words, nothing is going into the opioid receptors. When this happens everything hurts from sitting down to standing up, or just being touched. A draft of air that would normally be quite agreeable suddenly causes a chill. A meal causes cramps. A person suffering from withdrawal can temporarily become mentally unbalanced.

Luckily, withdrawal does not last forever. Within

a few days, the body once again begins to produce endorphins and things settle back to normal.

Endorphins must be encouraged in a pain situation. If you can learn to encourage the production of endorphins, you will lead a less painful life. You must not only learn to encourage endorphins, but also to eliminate the negative things that discourage the production of them.

The body has inherent ways to fight pain. It is important that you encourage these functions so your body has even more power. Where does this encouragement come from? Why, from your own brain.

:60 Second Brain Power

Remember:
1.	Your brain is the key component in fighting against pain.
2.	There is an old true saying, "No brain, no pain."
3.	Your brain tells you:
    •That you feel pain or pleasure
    •That you don't like the sensation of pain
    •The location of your pain
    •Whether this is like a pain you've had before or if this is a new pain
    •Whether the pain has increased
    or decreased
4.	Your brain also tries to decide what caused the pain, and what you can do about it.

The brain is not some omnipotent blob, but rather an intricately organized mass of cells. The brain has many centers of operation, and each center is responsible for something.

>•*AWARENESS CENTERS* tell us something
>is happening
>•*MEMORY CENTERS* are where long-term and
>short-term memories are stored
>•*LOCATION CENTERS* find where we have
>sensations on our body
>•*ACTION CENTERS* control action and all
>muscle movement
>•*CONTROL CENTERS* are responsible for our
>unique ability toward discipline, reason, and
>making decisions

Obviously, these mechanisms should not be hindered. All of these mechanisms are wonderfully elaborate and incredibly efficient. The lesson in the study of pain relief is that sometimes these mechanisms need encouragement.

Interference with pain-relieving systems can be due to many factors:

1. Prolonged narcotic use
2. Untreated depression
3. Pessimism
4. Inactivity, stiffening muscles

Pain is not just "in the head," but it can be treated there. Without your brain you would feel no pain, so don't shortchange your strongest weapon in the fight against chronic pain. Your body and brain both need treatment, as well as being actively involved in the management of pain.

:60 Second Pain Reality Check

Pain is real enough. So why is the validity of our pain sometimes questioned?

It is because we've all felt varying degrees of pain in our lives. There is an old saying, "My pain is real enough, but I don't know about yours."

There is a lot of truth to this old saying. It is common not to understand the pain of others, even others in our own family. Pain, especially chronic pain, is difficult to grasp if you do not suffer from it. Therefore, it is especially difficult for those who suffer from pain to get others to understand. Everyone reports their pain with different degrees of intensity. Pain can be imagined, but pain can also be real.

In the case of acute pain, its validity is not questioned. A toothache, a broken bone, a sore throat, or something obvious furnishes the physical proof that something is wrong. The reality of the pain is graphic in these scenarios.

Chronic pain is different, more complicated. You may or may not find a physical cause that explains the pain. Pain following a healed fracture, or a healed case of shingles, may show calluses in one case, or scars in the other, but nothing clearly explains why it hurts *now*.

Nevertheless, the pain is real. Just because the tests did not show any obvious reason for your pain does not mean the pain does not exist.

Somewhere in your nervous system there is a change that gives you the pain sensation. Attacking that change is often not easy. So it is with chronic pain.

However, you can change the way you feel about pain and the way it interferes with your lifestyle.

Of course, there are pains that are less "real." The malingerer makes up pain to avoid duty or work. Neurotic pains are a special group in which the patient seeks pain as punishment for some event in the past, as a form of atonement. The connection with a physical change cannot be found, because it is a psychological problem. People with severe psychosis sometimes complain of awful pains rather than talk of real underlying problems. This way of coping (or not coping) needs special treatment.

The degree to which pain is felt or reported varies from person to person. This does not mean one person's pain is more real than another's. The way we feel and report pain is partly a matter of how we learned to treat pain in our formative years. It also can depend on the training we receive in handling pain.

I believe you have the ability to control your pain responses. Your use of that ability is a great blessing for yourself and the people around you.

In other words, you don't have to be a pain to have a pain.

The Pain Experience

You know when you are in pain, or you may think you know. Whether or not you feel the pain at all partially depends on your mood, your activities at the time, and your outlook on life. Pain can be an all encompassing experience, as it is more than just physical.

By experiencing pain, you not only experience the physical sensation that comes with it, but what your mind does with it as well. *When pain is part of your consciousness, it is a pain experience.*

:60 Second Pain Update

•Some pains, especially acute ones, cannot be denied. Nor should they be denied.

•Your attitude regarding acute pain should be much different than your attitude concerning chronic pain.

•In experiencing acute pain, some action is called for and taken.

Chronic pain is different:

•Physical symptoms are often vague.

•Laboratory or x-ray results are not
always helpful.
•Whatever damage that has been done cannot
be undone.

In many cases, it is not something that is going to disappear. This is not easy to accept. Of course, you hope this pain will not last forever and that new treatments are being developed. But for now, assume that this chronic pain is something with which you have to live.

Live with it? This is not easy. The phrase can sound like an insult or an act of surrender from your doctor. If you don't know how to live with your pain, these seem to be cruel words.

But they are not cruel words, in fact, they are all kind words. Living with pain means *keeping the pain experience under control.* You can live with your pain.

But, in order to do so effectively, you must learn more about your condition. The irritation of a nerve root and the signal going along a nerve pathway are only part of the pain experience. What you think about pain, and how you feel when the pain occurs are the other aspects of the pain experience.

:60 Second Example—Dr. Lehndorff

> The point here is that there is a difference between giving up and modifying your activities.

I have had arthritis for thirty-five years. I've had

two hip operations for this condition. I've also had to change many things as a result—such as my way of walking. You may notice I did not say I suffered from it because that is precisely the point of this book. I want to put an end to suffering as much as possible.

Because of pains in my shoulder, I had to change my technique of playing the cello and piano. Notice, I did not say I gave them up. Instead, I modified the way I used my arms so I could continue with my passion for music.

My exercise program also had to change. I had to give up tennis. But I could still enjoy swimming, water-walking, stationary bicycling, and walking for exercise *and* pleasure.

Since my way of walking had to be modified, I can no longer go on the fast and long hikes I used to enjoy. I now enjoy short walks using a cane where I commune with the trees, the flowers, and the seasons. I've also continued my hobby of teaching lifesaving. I just teach from a sitting position now.

I also have a heart problem and a stomach ulcer. These caused me to give up other things, risky things. I quit smoking, gave up caffeine, and lost seventy-five pounds.

Time and Pain

Leon, in his early sixties, had an operation for cancer of the tongue. Part of his jaw had to be removed, and the nerve that provides the sensory function for the tongue had to be cut.

In that nerve, the patient experienced severe, sudden stabbing pains. He described the pain as "like lightening." He meant that the pain came on very fast, was very intense, and then disappeared quickly. Leon was especially bothered by the fact that he could never predict when the pain was going to happen, or how often it would occur.

Remember:
•Some pains come and go.
•Some pains stay a short time.
•Some pains keep coming back.

:60 Second Pain Information

•Spasms have a rhythm.
•Stabs of pain are unpredictable.

The concept of time influences our perception of pain. It may increase or diminish the suffering that accompanies the pain. While acute pain is difficult to bear, you can frequently predict how long the pain will last. This can help a bad situation.

With chronic pain, it is much more difficult to predict the length of pain. In arthritis or lower back-ache, there are certain activities that tend to aggravate the pain, but remember many are still possible to enjoy.

The key is that you must learn to pace yourself. Pacing is a time-related activity. You must divide your daily exercises into small segments spread across the day. This way you can use time for your own benefit.

Chapter 2

You and
Your Pain

There is a difference between pain and suffering.
If you do an exercise that you have not done in a long time, you may feel pain in your muscles. However, even if you become stiff and sore, you will feel proud and be pleased with yourself. Exercise is good for you. This pain is what athletes rightfully call "good pain."

The separation regarding pain and suffering may be illustrated by the attitude of some women toward childbirth. Their level of pain depends on many things:

1. It depends on cultural influences.
2. Their attitude toward the child to be borne.
3. The training they received in pain management.
4. The particular birth.
5. Complications.

In Lamaze training, there are techniques taught in order to focus on the good part of this experience. I have found that many of those techniques have universal applications for pain other than those of childbirth.

:60 Second Childbirth Applications

---

1.   The power of words; just using the expression "contraction" instead of "pain" makes a huge difference.
2.   Proper breathing techniques reduce stress and pain at the same time.
3.   The trained participation of the husband eliminates a great deal of anxiety.
4.   The positive aspect of the experience is stressed, helping reduce some of the anxiety and suffering.

Remember, almost all women have discomfort or pain in childbirth, but not all suffer.

Complaining Constantly, Suffering Silently

:60 Second People Questions

One of the problems you face with chronic pain is whether or not you let people know how you feel.

•Do you tell people the details?
•Do you tell a person about the pain every time

you see them?
•Do people want to know?
•Should you suffer in silence?

There is a middle ground. Suffering in silence is not good. You know that, maybe all too well. It may lead to a martyr complex. That certainly does not contribute to your improvement. If you tell people about your pain, try to separate descriptions of the pain from how you feel about it. For example, you could say, "This sharp pain in my back has made it so hard for me to move that it interferes with some of the things I want to do." This is a good way to think of your pain experience because it is positive. This way you are not denying reality, but rather separating your mental reactions to the pain from the description of pain.

:60 Second Attitude Advice:

•Open your mind to a helpful attitude. An attitude of persevering, not of suffering.
•React to the pain in ways to influence your pain perception.
•Remember, feelings regarding pain are often more open to improvement than the pain sensation is.

As simple as this sounds, an utterance denoting a positive attitude can help.

:60 Second Pain Improvement Sound Bytes

•The pain is there but I don't seem to mind it so much today.
•The pain is there but I'm too busy to bother with it.
•I love my job! I won't let pain interfere with it!
•This is a beautiful day and just looking at it makes me feel I can forget my pain for a while.

When you can say these statements with regularity and sincerity, you have begun to cope.

:60 Seconds at a Time

It is important to understand how time is lived. Some people live their lives in terms of years or larger chunks of time. Others in terms of months, or weeks. But if you are in chronic pain and think in these time segments, it's easy to get frustrated. This occurs because either it may have been years since you didn't feel pain or you could become very depressed about what your thoughts of the future encompass.

It doesn't have to be this way.

In fact, try a new way of thinking, a :60 second way of thinking. Don't think of time in huge, unmanageable chunks.

:60 Second Way of Thinking

Try to forget your pain for :60 second periods:
During this period, try something else such as:
1. Smiling.
2. Taking an interest in something.
3. Asking someone else how they feel, then, in the next :60 second interval, think about how their answer made you feel.

Food for Thought

It is very important to eat healthy, nutritious food, especially if you are experiencing chronic pain. Not only does proper nutrition play a significant part in healing, but if you are taking medication, nutrition becomes even more important.

Moderation, good judgement, and proper planning can improve your diet. Your general health is even more important than pain control, and that is why diet is so important.

A proper daily diet should follow the food pyramid published by the government. At the top, on the smallest part of the pyramid, are listed fats and sweets. The use of saturated fats, such as butter, have certain dangers. Polyunsaturated fats are safer to use. Olive oil is an example of a polyunsaturated fat.

Milk, yogurt, and cheese should be treated with respect. Calcium is an important nutrient. However, getting it from high cholesterol-containing foods should be avoided or used in moderation. For example, most adults can get an adequate supply of calcium from skim milk and avoid the fat of whole milk and high-fat cheeses.

Protein sources include meat, poultry, fish, dry beans, eggs, and nuts. Protein is needed for a healthy diet. Fat is not. Cut down your consumption of meat and when you have it, choose lean cuts; trim all fat. Remove chicken skin and go easy on eggs, especially egg yolks.

Dark green vegetables are good vitamin and mineral sources, as are deep yellow vegetables, dry beans, and legumes. Eating them, as well as salads, will provide needed roughage, vitamins, and minerals. Fruits are also an essential source of roughage, vitamins, and minerals.

Rice, cereals, breads, and pasta are at the bottom of the pyramid. Try to get whole grain products whenever possible.

As for quantities, it is better to eat five small meals a day than to consume massive calories at one big meal.

Vitamins

Vitamins are essential for life and health. They occur in the body in small amounts, yet the small amounts of these substances are powerful and useful. If a needed vitamin is missing from your diet, illnesses of various kinds may occur.

However, these substances must be treated with respect because it is possible to overdose. Generally, if you eat a balanced diet, you will get all the vitamins that you need. It is usually not necessary to take vitamin supplements unless they are prescribed for certain medical conditions or dietary lacks. However, a multivitamin capsule may have benefits and will not be harmful.

Recently, there has been a lot written about antioxidants to correct certain conditions. Nevertheless, research is still preliminary. Not enough has been published in medical journals, while too much has been published in public journals and the daily press. Vitamins C and E, as well as Beta Carotene, may act as antioxidants.

Essentially, antioxidants interfere with the oxidation of certain substances in the body. When these substances are oxidated in the body, they can present a health hazard. For example, oxidation of LDL cholesterol particles may be an important step in the formation of arterial plaques. As the results of more long-term studies become available, the true value of antioxidants will be revealed.

I would like to stress that lifestyle plays a more vital role in preventing disease than vitamin therapy. Although vitamin research is promising, it is more important not to smoke, to control diabetes and high blood pressure, exercise, control weight, and eat a proper diet.

Vitamin capsules are not a substitute for choosing healthy foods to eat.

Your Mood and Your Pain

Everyone has "good" days and "bad" days. Everybody also has mood swings from "up" (elated) to "down" (depressed). Moderate changes in mood are perfectly normal, but excessive mood swings need to be corrected.

:60 Second "Suffering Thoughts"
to Watch Out for:

1.	Nobody understands me, they can't imagine how badly I feel.
2.	I'll never lead a normal life.
3.	This is humiliating.
4.	I can't do what I used to do.
5.	I am sad and discouraged.
6.	My sadness is so deep and long-lasting that I can't imagine anyone helping me.

There are many more negative thoughts of course. None are helpful. They are all self-defeating. Remember, the mind has immense powers. The mind has powers over the chemical workings of your nervous system.

If you are seriously depressed, medical help is available. It is essential to cleanse the mind before proceeding in your quest for a more vibrant life.

:60 Second Positive Answers to Negative Thoughts

> 1.   I will stop worrying whether anyone understands me. From now on, I'll try to understand others--one person at a time, :60 seconds at a time.
> 2.   I will lead an effective, useful life. It will be different from my present lifestyle. I will live in short, paced intervals. I will live!
> 3.   If I make an effort and fail, I will not be humiliated. I will consider it a challenge to meet next time.

Linda's Depression

Linda was a former ice skater who had severe leg and back pain because of a fall and had to quit a promising career.

Fortunately, several methods of treatment worked for Linda. She responded well to muscle relaxants. She also derived great benefit from techniques such as relaxation response and visual imagery which you will learn about later (Chapter 4).

In fact, Linda responded so well to exercises that she was able to avoid injections most of the time.

There was only one problem. About twice a year, Linda went into a deep depression that she had to be treated for. In fact, it became clear that she would not respond to any medical treatment until she pulled out of her mental depression. Once she was depression—free for a few weeks, the medical treatments for her condition were effective again.

The :60 second lesson here is quite simple. For better or worse, the mind can act as a strong force on the condition of the body.

Busman's Backache

Charles is a bus driver who suffered a back injury some years before. He had backaches, and he asked me for help because these backaches were threatening to interfere with his job.

Charles drove the bus on long trips for tour groups. He would drive people from Massachusetts to Montreal, or to places all over the Northeast. On these trips, Charles' body got stiff, even though he felt the driving was easy.

Luggage also presented a problem. The job required his getting luggage in and out of the luggage carriers. Thus, further aggravating the back strain.

Most of the passengers on his trips were golden agers and needed assistance. Longer trips had more overnight stays, thus there were more bags and more handling of luggage.

The day Charles came to my office he did not have any pain, but he knew it would return. We discussed more efficient ways of driving buses to prevent strain. Then, I brought up the possibility of giving up longer trips which required him to handle luggage.

"Do shorter routes, I suggested."

"Oh no. I love my job," he declared. "I enjoy the trips, the fun, and the friendly atmosphere."

We worked out some adjustments which would allow him to continue working because he liked what he was doing. There is no limit to the kind of adjustments we can make when we have a job we love.

Spontaneous Improvement

Is it possible for pain to stop all by itself? In my records, there are a number of people whose disability improvements cannot be explained by standard good treatment alone. The improvement is due to something else. I tried to figure out the causes.

A number of patients who improved dramatically had strong religious beliefs. These patients believed there was a connection between their improvement and faith.

The term "faith factor" was coined by Dr. Herbert Benson, director of the Mind/Body Institute at

Deaconess Hospital in Boston, and a Professor of
Medicine at Harvard University Medical School. Dr.
Benson believes that the faith factor has strong medical
implications. It is the only thing that will explain some
startling examples of recovery or improvement. The
faith factor is not associated with any particular religion.

:60 Second Faith Factors:

Faith comes into play when you believe in something. This may be belief in your doctor, your medicines,
your exercises, and, most of all, yourself. By having faith,
you increase your possibilities of improvement. In fact,
faith may actually facilitate some chemical changes in
your body that help fight pain, stress, and depression.
Religious belief can be especially important.

Faith can also discourage the body's production of
harmful substances that tend to increase pain, stress, and
depression.

Believe it.

Sympathy and Sickness

When you have pain, you want others to understand what you are feeling. This is only natural.

Unfortunately, the display of sympathy has some
undesirable side reactions. Instead of making you feel
better, an overt show of sympathy may make you feel

weak and helpless.

You may think, "I must be in terrible shape because everybody looks so sad and concerned when they see me."

The better message for people to convey is that they understand that you are sick, but that they believe in your strength to rebound. The message should exude confidence that you will fight your way out of your situation.

In most situations, the best thing to do while you are enduring pain is to continue doing everything you are capable of. Try letting go of those things you are not. This may not be easy, but this kind of honesty allows others to deal with you honestly. When you regain confidence in yourself, others will too.

:60 Second Victory and Defeat Messages

You cannot win them all. This is true.

However, you can win some of life's battles. Life has not beaten you. When things do not work out your way, you are not defeated. When things went wrong for England in World War II and London was bombed, Winston Churchill said, "Never give up. Never give up. Never ever give up."

Keep trying. Yes, sometimes you will lose, but you already have the personal victory of your effort. Moreover, there are other victories you can win: self-esteem victories, health victories, and joy victories. Life, after all, is still life.

•Any time you *do something* that you don't particularly feel like doing but know is good for you, it is a victory. It is an accomplishment achieved by small steps taken :60 seconds at a time.

•Anytime you *omit something* that you know to be bad for you is another victory.

•Everyday, you can live little victories and build toward larger goals. By *winning little skirmishes* with your body or your mood, you prepare yourself for a life where pain is not your primary focus.

Victory *can* begin in :60 second segments.

Litigation, Settlements, and Pain

People who are in pain have been frequently involved in an accident at work, in the car, or in leisure activities. Therefore, with chronic pain often comes litigation.

Litigation is strong medicine, and like all strong medicine, it has side reactions. Despite your suffering, a pain clinic or pain doctor will try to teach you to start living with your pain. The clinic will teach you to ignore the pain as much as possible. Remember, *pain gets worse with the amount of attention paid to it*.

However, the legal situation is very different, almost opposite. You have to prove your claim and by doing so, it is natural that you pay a lot of attention to your pain. Thus, it is very difficult to employ the exercises you would normally use in fighting pain.

If you have to demonstrate suffering to get a good settlement, you are giving yourself a powerful suggestion, and suggestions can be used for many purposes. This is not about being honest or dishonest. Rather, it is about your basic humanity and the way your brain works. For better or worse, your mind is stronger than your body.

Having studied pain for decades, I know that many people have remarkable changes in their conditions once lawsuits are settled. Afterward, the part of pain that is aggravated by the stress of litigation often vanishes.

Consider the story of Julio, a man in his late twenties, who worked in the construction industry. I treated Julio whose serious injuries were incurred when a pile of bricks had fallen on top of him. We used a variety of methods, but nothing seemed to work.

Then one day, he reported to me that his most recent set of injections had helped. He told me that his medication had pulled him out of his depression. He also said that his diet was working, and he was losing the weight he needed in order to move more efficiently.

Immediately, I noticed an enormous change in Julio. He had gone from passive sufferer to active fighter. The difference was astonishing. Naturally, I was curious as to what brought about these changes. The answer was that he had recently settled his lawsuit.

Override

When the mind and body are kept busy to the extent that pain is not perceived or noticed, it is called "override."

Override succeeds.

The brain works like a computer, or perhaps we should say that a computer works like a brain. The brain (or the computer) can only handle one problem at a time. Some people would say that they do a million things at one time. This is an illusion. In fact, when you concentrate, you force your mind to work on only one thing.

Override works best when there are strong emotional overtones in your thought processes. Anything of great personal interest will cause override. So will fear, danger, and ambition. Anything that moves you strongly causes override. The feelings can be positive or negative, but they must be strong feelings. If you are consumed with something else, your pain is pushed to the background.

Override works. Here are some examples:

:60 Second Override Examples

1.   Bob came to me complaining of pain from post herpetic neuralgia. This is chronic pain which occurs after an attack of shingles. When we started discussing his life and his pain, it became clear that he was

a very busy man.

He runs a small electronics firm. He teaches physics at MIT as well, and he even sometimes ventures to Europe to give lectures on particle physics.

Bob told me, "When I teach or when I work, I feel no pain."

But Bob also said when he sat down at the end of a busy day, he felt considerable pain.

I asked him if he had hobbies.

He shook his head. "I used to write poetry," he confessed, "but I'm too busy."

I suggested that he try writing poetry again during his free time. Bob did, and showed me the poems. He was a very talented writer.

When I asked Bob how he felt while writing the poems, he answered, "I wasn't paying attention to my pain at those times."
Override works.

2.   Denise, a middle-aged woman, came to me because she was experiencing frequent and painful backaches. However, she confessed that for four hours on Sunday afternoons, she had no pain. On that day, she had a table at which she sold antiques at a big flea market in Hollis, New Hampshire.

During those four hours, she bought, sold, wrapped, and picked up packages. She bent and stretched. She had a wonderful time talking to those at the tables around hers.

Override works.

3.   Another woman, Harriet, had a hunch-
back and was in her seventies when she came to me,
complaining of considerable back, rib, and arm pains
from osteoporosis. Her bones were very brittle. She had
fractured two vertebrae.

Despite this, twice a week for three hours in the
evening, she played bingo. She experienced no pain
during that time. Bingo? Yes, bingo. She played eight
cards at a time.

Imagine the motion. Reaching and moving to
eight cards, and concentrating on the numbers called.
And, of course, turning and twisting as she laughed and
talked with those around her.
Override works.

4.   During the Italian campaign of World
War II, a beach head was established near Anzio. The
area was wide but not very deep. Thus, every wounded
soldier could be moved to a hospital ship in a relatively
short time.

A study was done on how these soldiers reacted to
different types of treatment. Some of the soldiers who
were wounded received the standard treatment given by
the Army Medical Corps. First, a medical soldier who
found the wounded man would give him an injection of
morphine so the victim could be transported without too
much discomfort. The next step would be bringing him

to the Battalion Aid Station, and then the Collection Station, the Clearing Station, and finally, a boat would transport him to the hospital ship. At each of these stops, if the patient complained of pain, more medication was given. They all complained of pain.

Some wounded soldiers were treated differently. They were told truthfully and emphatically that they would be brought to the hospital ship quickly and that everything would be done to repair the damage of their wound. And they were told that if the situation demanded prolonged recovery, the soldier would be shipped home for further care.

The interesting point is that the soldiers in the second group required only a fraction of the pain medication of the first group. They were less anxious. They were reassured every step of the way. They had less anxiety, and less pain.

If you help your mind, you can help your body.

5.   One study was done on surgery patients by Dr. Lawrence Egbert of Massachusetts General Hospital. He analyzed the pre-anesthetic preparation of patients, in other words the interviews with patients before surgery.

Half the patients were interviewed in a routine way during which they were told what the surgery was and what kind of anesthetic would be used.

The other half had more elaborate interviews. Those patients were told they would go to sleep easily

or be numbed adequately. They were assured they
would not feel pain during the operation. It was also
explained that after surgery, they would wake up com-
fortably in the Recovery Room and remain that way.

The patients who had more elaborate interviews
and who were given reassuring information experienced
much less pain. They needed less pain-relieving
medication than the group who had standard interviews.
These people had a great deal less nausea; they got out
of bed quicker, left the hospital sooner, and resumed
normal lives earlier.

Predicting Improvement

You can predict improvement. No, that does not
mean a cure. Improvement means that some aspect of
your situation is about to get better or is already
getting better.

The markers on the road are there if you just look.
Look for a decrease in pain, improved quality of life,
and especially, the ability to do more.

The will to improve is a vital key to success. If
you have an iron will to improve, then the treatments
the doctor prescribe are likely to work. The treatment,
of course, must be selected for the individual patient
with some care:

:60 Second Criteria for High Possibility of Improvement

1.	Weight loss, if required (slow and gradual)
2.	Caffeine reduction (when suggested)
3.	Smoking reduction or cessation
4.	"Down" time reduced, "up" time increased
5.	Exercise resumed

Here are some indicators of good probability of improvement:

1. Resumption of attendance at religious service
2. Resumption of social activities
3. Participation in a support group

:60 Second Visualization

1.	Picture the area of your pain.
2.	Picture an area around the pain center that has a greater sensitivity to touch.
3.	Picture both areas a little bit smaller. Just a little.
4.	Picture both areas getting smaller. Every :60 seconds, try and shrink the area pictured in your mind just a little. See how far you can shrink it.

Make a New Start

You have traveled the route. You have seen a number of doctors, maybe a surgeon. You have had physiotherapy, taken drugs, and seen more doctors. Maybe you've tried a chiropractor. So, why are you still experiencing pain?

Unless you are one of the fortunate people for whom medical or surgical intervention is completely successful, afterward you are probably about where you were before—still in pain.

There is one more person who might be able to help you. In fact, this person *can* help you. Probably, this person has never been a full-fledged member of your medical care team.

It is time to bring that person on board.

That person is *you.*

It is not easy to become directly involved in your own improvement, but it is essential. You will be amazed at what you can do if you can learn to unleash the powers of your mind. The miracles that you perform must be done in small installments, that's the secret.

Remember, you are not helpless. There is enormous untapped strength within you. You just have to learn to mobilize that power. It takes practice. It will not happen overnight. But improvement can and will happen if you put your mind to it.

Change is only :60 seconds away.

:60 Second New Start Ideas

1.   Tell yourself clearly: "I want to get better. I can get better. I will get better."
2.   Pick an easy interim goal and plan for it. It should be something you like to do, perhaps a short walk.
3.   Try a hobby you have not done in a while. It could be playing a musical instrument, or some sort of craft. Don't overextend, but give it a ten-minute try as a first step.
4.   Write a letter to a friend who has not heard from you in a while.
5.   Try something a bit more difficult. Try some exercises you have neglected. Perhaps you will have to break the execution of these into parts at the beginning. Don't get discouraged; celebrate partial success as a breakthrough.
6.   Keep a journal for the day and write down every extra thing you accomplished.
7.   Look for little bits of improvement. Keep a list of these.
8.   If you find a paragraph in this book you find helpful, copy it on an index card. Look at it a few times a day as an affirmation.
9.   Remember that the most important person on your health care team looks at you every day from your mirror.
10.   When you look in the mirror, tell yourself today you will improve.

Chapter 3

Using Your Pain

One of the most troubling beliefs found in chronic pain patients is that they were selected for punishment by a higher power. It is a hard belief to abandon.

It is a common answer to the question, Why me?

After all, when you have chronic pain, such a question could be on your mind often.

The answer is not clear. Most religions promise rewards after death but they are not as explicit about rewards or punishments in *this* life. But many teach or insinuate that leading the right life means having a good life.

Yet there is a certain randomness built into the cycle of life. Most people lead average lives. But on the extremes of the statistical curve, you find pain, illness, and failure on one side. And on the other? Miracles and unexpected good luck.

We have certainly not been able to relate

sickness to health in any but statistical ways. There are no absolutes.

Therefore, the question is still unanswered and the "why me" feeling persists. Nevertheless, no matter who you are, you were not selected for punishment. Perhaps you are being tested.

An old cliche which is still useful is: "Fate handed you a lemon, so make some lemonade."

Think of a runner in the Boston Marathon. The runner accomplishes little by complaining about the famous Heartbreak Hill. The runner knows the hill is there. If the runner wants to run in the Boston Marathon, he has to deal with it. He has to train differently, adjusting his physical conditioning with uphill runs, and adjusting his attitude towards struggle and pain.

This is not minor pain that these runners experience. On Heartbreak Hill, the runners accumulate acid in their muscles, causing pain, especially in their calf muscles. Then the endorphins kick in. The body begins to produce these pain-fighting chemicals, and the runner can fight his/her way to the top.

Obviously, if you, like the runner, could produce endorphins to fight your pain you would benefit. You can. It can be done by electronic stimulation, acupuncture, hypnosis, and especially exercise.

There is no need to run a marathon. Just learn from those who do. Endorphins help in the fight against pain. So try to make a few endorphins every day.

If Only I Had No Pain

Have you ever caught yourself thinking, "If only
. . ." For instance, if only I had no pain, I could do this
or that. If only I had no pain, I could go back to work,
for a long walk or exercise. If only I had less pain, I
would be less tense. I would be kinder to my family.

These are not idle hopes. They are good long-
range goals. They are unsuitable only if you desire them
as short-term plans. In fact, this thought process is more
appropriate for acute pain, which stops you from using
the part of your body that is diseased or damaged.

Chronic pain is different. By the time the pain has
lasted long enough to be diagnosed as chronic, your
habits have changed. Your new habits may actually
aggravate the pain.

It is important to understand that if you stick with
any one activity for a long time, you may aggravate the
pain sensation. However, if you sit still or rest for too
long you will get stiff, inelastic muscles that can also
aggravate the pain sensation.

You need a different approach.

:60 Second Planning

•You need to do some planning. Some specific planning not just for the indefinite future, but for the next day.
•Plan the next hour. Plan the next :60 seconds!
•Plan things you can do.
•Throw in a minor challenge from time to time.
•Any minute spent in some form of activity will contribute to your improvement.

It won't always be easy and sometimes you will have to force yourself, just like the runners in the Boston Marathon. But if you force yourself to do it, it is a victory. And no small victory.

Your Plan:

:60 Second Limitation Rules

•Don't pretend you do not have limitations. You know you do, so don't fool yourself.
•Acknowledge your limitations. And then *limit your limitations.*
•Take them in stride and do things with purpose.
•When you rest, do it to get ready for some later activity or in order to recover from doing some thing demanding.
•Plan your rest periods. During the day, it is better to rest frequently rather than for a long period.

Plan other activities as well. For instance, if you walk, plan ahead of time how far you will walk. Don't go beyond your limits, but think of today's limit as temporary. Tomorrow set new, slightly higher ones.

Take control of your life. Stop saying, "If only I didn't have pain, I could do things." Instead, think of the things you will be able to do if you control your pain.

Once you start thinking positively, you are on the road to success. Soon, you will be doing things that you once thought impossible.

How to Use Your Pain

Constant pain seems to those enduring it debilitating and useless.

Acute pain, of course, is different. It tells us that something immediate is wrong; a broken nose, appendicitis, a throat infection, or any of a million other things. Acute pain is a warning and serves a valuable purpose. A broken bone hurts less when properly splinted, and a sore throat is a warning that a person must get proper medical treatment. That is the theory.

However, chronic pain defies that theory. Chronic pain sticks around even though there is no further damage to the tissue or organ. The damage is already done.

In some cases of chronic pain, there is no obvious sign of tissue damage. Does that mean there is no pain?

No, there is pain. You feel it. In fact, there are ways to find where this pain registers. It could register under the skin, in the nerves, in the joints, in the spinal cord, or even in some small memory centers in the brain.

However, such pain is useless in all ways except one. The brain is your weapon in the battle against pain. That's right, you can use your brain to fight your pain.

Chronic pain indicates clearly that you must make certain changes in your life and lifestyle. Some changes of which we've already spoken are quite obvious. For instance, pain in the back, legs, lower joints, or lower half of the body can be aggravated by excess weight. Obviously, a step to take is to get body weight back to normal or even slightly below normal for your height.

Exercise is another method of alleviating pain. You do not want to do an overreaching program of exercise, but rather exercise that gives you a slight ache. Remember, a slight ache, good pain, is healthy.

The ache gives feedback to tell you that you have done enough exercise for the moment. Stop and return to the exercises later, or even the next day. When you begin exercising again, you should continue until you feel an ache.

Walking is a good example. It would be ideal if you could walk four miles every day without stopping, but, many people in chronic pain cannot do that. Certainly not when they begin extended walking for the first time.

If you can walk ten minutes without too much pain, you should adjust your walking program to that. You could walk away from your house five minutes in one direction, turn around and walk back. If you do that six times a day, that's a total of one hour walked! That's just as good (and perhaps better for you!) than if you had walked the entire distance in one session.

This strategy works the same way for all exercises such as swimming, aerobics, or riding a bike—stationary or mobile.

:60 Second Strategies Activity

- The key is to *pace yourself.*
- Change positions.
- Change activities.
- Rest or end your rest.
- Figure out a way to make things work for you.
- If you use a typewriter or computer, you may have to adjust your position.
- The important thing to adjust is your attitude.
- If you want to do something within reason, you will.

The Incredible Power of the Mind

The mind is more powerful than the body. The mind can will the body to perform certain actions. If I think: Move my left arm, my left arm will move.

You can alter even some of the functions that are automatic with your mind. You can change your breathing, pulse rate, and blood pressure if you train your mind to do these things.

However, it is a sad truth that the condition of your body can influence your mood too. It can sometimes override logical thinking.

Your moods are powerful. You may feel happy because you had a good breakfast, or perhaps displeased because you ate too much. You can feel unhappy because you have pain, or happy because you have none. You can aggravate your pain if you are depressed, or you can reduce your pain if you feel happy about something.

You can certainly override your pain if you are in danger and try to escape. You can forget your pain if you are challenged by an important issue.

The strength of the mind is like the strength of a muscle. If you want a muscle to be strong, you don't just expect normal use of that muscle to do it. You devise artificial means called exercise. If you exercise a muscle enough, it becomes stronger. You must also exercise your mind to give it the strength to win your battle against chronic pain.

Another consideration when thinking about the power of the mind is that the power of the mind is intensified when there is an emotional hook. For example, if your life is endangered, you are probably not too concerned about your pain at that time. Likewise, if you are happy about some success, you can postpone your pain for a bit.

Enjoyment, fear, danger, and success all have strong emotional overtones. *You can learn to use your brain to fight your pain.*

Thoughts on Learning

Many people with chronic pain have a lot of time on their hands. They may feel they cannot work. They may have been told their jobs are too strenuous or stressful. Staying home, staring at the television and feeling sorry for themselves, time can quickly become an enemy for these people. Unless some activities are added, time will add to the pain by the mere opportunity to dwell upon it.

There is truth to this statement made by a woman in a television commercial: "I haven't got time for the pain." When the actress says this, she is referring to override, which was discussed earlier. The truth is, time must be occupied in order to help you forget about the pain.

One of the best ways to fill available time is to learn a hobby. There may even be things that you always wanted to study but didn't have the time. Now you have time. So use it.

Just remember that your approach to learning may have to be a bit different than it was in the past. You may have to stop more frequently and rest. You may also have to take your time learning. There's nothing wrong with that.

If your pain has caused you to change jobs or even temporarily quit working, learning is even more important. You may need a job that is less physically demanding than your last one. In that case, it could be more mentally challenging and you may need more education. Many jobs involve computers. If you are over thirty, you may not have had computer training. This is a good time to begin learning to operate a computer.

Using one means primarily engaging the mind and not the body.

However, remember that your training process should be planned at a slower pace because of your pain.

Pacing

Erin was in her early forties when she had a terrible automobile accident causing severe brain damage and a fractured vertebra. It was a very difficult time but she lived through it. She underwent an operation which required stabilizing rods in her back and extensive therapy: speech therapy, physiotherapy, occupational therapy, and psychotherapy.

Erin is now able to function quite well but still has frequent episodes of considerable back pain. It is a difficult situation but Erin has made it worse by being unable to pace herself. She is overly conscientious. Everything she starts must be finished without rest and without regard to whether she is in pain or not. "I've got to finish things," Erin says when asked about this compulsive habit.

Erin stubbornly refused to learn from her pain. Instead of working with her pain, she worked against it. This only makes her life more difficult.

The lesson to be learned from Erin's story is that you must pace yourself. Do not demand of yourself, as Erin did, that you complete things as quickly as you once did. When you learn to pace yourself, you can make your life better.

:60 Second Pacing Plan

1.	Do things in *short installments*.
2.	Rest in short installments.
3.	Vary your activities and keep going.
4.	Don't give up but don't overextend.

Remember: Even *small steps are big steps*. If you don't want to try an activity because you fear it, *pretend* you can do it. Once you begin, *the sense of accomplishment will far outweigh the pain.*

Keep Moving

One of the big fears with chronic pain is the fear of motion. You think it will hurt if you move. This is only partly true. The full truth is that if you don't move, it will hurt even more.

For those with a religious orientation, there is an old saying: "Pray as though you could do nothing by yourself, and work as though there were no higher power to help you." However you approach this task, don't give up. Keep moving, keep doing.

:60 Second Rules for Moving

> If sitting bothers you, STAND UP.
> If standing bothers you, SIT DOWN.
> If sitting still bothers you, WALK AROUND.
> If walking bothers you, SIT DOWN.
> If being glum bothers you, SMILE.
> If smiling bothers you, LAUGH.
> If laughing bothers you, REALLY? DOES IT?

It is certainly easy to deny these rules with the thought that you are not in the mood. That's possible. But that's such an easy exercise. Try again. This time, pretend you are in the mood. Trick yourself. Keep pretending.

Remember to do things in short intervals. If you do housework, you do not have to finish it all at once. You can rest, and while you are, you can occupy your mind with reading or a craft or something else that interests you.

There is a lesson we can learn from people who lived in the eighteenth and early nineteenth centuries. During those periods, people had desks for sitting and separate desks for standing. When people got tired of sitting, they just stood up, moved to their other desks, and continued with their paperwork. And when they tired of working while standing, they sat down.

If you are a clock watcher, this system works well. You can time any activity and learn to stop before it causes you real pain. A little ache, of course, is quite acceptable. If you can establish a routine where you make yourself get up and do more, you will feel better about yourself. When you make your body obey this new command, even for short intervals, you have succeeded!

There is a difference between up time and down time. Down time is spent sleeping, sitting, or lounging. There is nothing wrong with down time within certain limits.

Up time keeps us active. It does not have to be strenuous activity such as running or weight lifting. A short walk may be enough of a beginning. Just do a series of short walks. Pace yourself.

:60 Second Time Keeper

---

1.   Regulate your down time and up time by simply keeping track of both in a notebook.

2.   Tally both items at the end of each day.

3.   See if you can increase your up time by a small amount each day. When you do, you are on your way to improvement.

To illustrate this philosophy compare active endeavors to inactive endeavors. For example, a short swim is better for you than a long sit in a whirlpool. Likewise a short walk has more benefits than a long massage. Granted, the whirlpool and massage have some benefits, but anytime you do something for yourself, the benefits to body and soul are greater.

Anything you do actively is more valuable than anything that is done to you or for you. We ask people, what did you do today? We do not ask, how long did you sit and wait for things to happen to you today?

Help and Helpfulness

It is important to do things for others as well as for yourself. It is essential for your self-esteem. When you have given something of yourself to someone else, your relations with others will improve.

You may ask how can you possibly help someone else when you are in such pain? You may even ask whom you could possibly help? The answer is simple.

First, you will help yourself. Remember, anytime you do something for someone else, you are also helping yourself. That is one reason why support groups are so important.

In a support group, people learn they are not alone. You may have found a way to cope with some aspect of your pain and you can share it. You can learn from others and you can offer support.

It's the same in other situations. You may not be able to carry big packages for someone, but even carrying something small can be helpful if a person has their hands full. Little things are a big help, both to those you help and to yourself for obvious reasons of self esteem. Just offering a sympathetic ear to someone can be one of the finest things you can do for another person.

Thoughts On Gratitude

Things may look bleak. But maybe you haven't looked close enough. There is an exercise you can do, well-known in psychological circles, that is helpful in realizing things are not so terrible after all.

:60 Second Thankfulness List

1.	Everyday, make a list of things you are thankful for. Start with a list of three things.
2.	Increase the list by one each day.
3.	Repeat the items you listed on the previous day.
4.	Get as creative and outrageous as you would like.

You can be thankful that the sun is shining or you can be thankful that it is a cool, cloudy day. You may be happy that your favorite team won, that a neighbor had some good fortune, or that a relative received a job promotion.

Impress yourself that you were able to exercise or walk a bit longer than you did the previous day. Be happy when you hear a favorite song on the radio or see an enjoyable show on television. Be glad you are alive. Be grateful you have a roof over your head. No matter what, keep that list going.

Remember, the more time you spend on these positive things, the less time you will have to dwell on negative thoughts of pain.

Chapter 4

Good and
Bad Stress

A man and a woman who do not know each other are walking through a crowded public square when suddenly their eyes meet. If this man and this woman are attracted to each other, both of them feel something happen at that moment, not just to their eyes, but throughout their bodies. However, added to the immediate feeling of attraction is another feeling, stress.

All the signs are there. Pulse rates and blood pressure go up. Blood sugars rise. Adrenaline increases and muscle tone improves. Both people are experiencing stress, all right. But is it bad? Hardly.

In fact, your body often produces a healthy level of stress at just the opportune moment. For instance, if you have to give a public speech your body will undergo many of the same changes, essentially revving you up so you will give a great speech. Like the stress of the two people attracted to each other, the feeling is not a bad one.

Good Stress

Stress, despite the ominous sound to the word, is actually a good biological response to a situation. As stated above, it occurs in romance, but it also occurs in other situations as well.

It is important to understand that stress serves a purpose. It is, in a sense, part of the body's defense mechanisms—often referred to as the "fight-or-flight" reaction. This is called acute stress. I like to refer to it as good stress because it is, in fact, good. It makes the body ready for a challenge.

For example, you are on a leisurely drive, suddenly a car swerves into your lane and you almost have an accident. Notice that your body has undergone many split-second changes. You become more alert as adrenaline is pumped into the blood stream. Additionally, blood pressure and pulse are increased. Blood sugar also rises, bringing sugar to the muscles and brain. All of these reactions serve a purpose, to get the body and the brain ready for immediate action. The body reacts to a fight-or-flight situation.

The same thing occurs more gradually as you prepare for something like a test or a public speaking engagement. The challenge causes those changes.

Another example of good stress is when you do

an aerobic exercise. The body understands your need for more energy and it makes the proper adjustments.

In fact, in a healthy person, stress is a lifesaving reflex for specific situations. These acute stress reactions diminish when the situation fades.

Bad Stress

There is another kind of stress, of course, the kind that has given the word such a bad name. If you are "stressed out," you understand.

Bad stress is the kind that doesn't go away. In other words, it is chronic. It happens like this: You perceive a danger, just as in acute stress. The danger is not a specific situation, but rather a predicament of some sort. It is seemingly beyond your control and has caused the same biological changes in your body as acute stress.

However, the difference is that the predicament, whether it be an overbearing boss, a challenging job, a difficult marriage, or even a past danger (post traumatic stress), is ongoing and therefore so is the stress. The body, essentially, does not return to a relaxation mode. With chronic stress, it is normal always to be on the alert. And that is bad.

To understand the difference between acute and chronic stress, imagine a blaring fire siren. If you hear it, you know there is some sort of emergency and some action must be taken. The siren produces acute stress.

Now imagine that the fire is out and somehow the siren got stuck. It blares on and on, over and over. It is, of course, no less loud; almost sounding louder, even though logic tells you it is at the same level. It just roars and roars and you want it to stop, because it is so annoying and uncomfortable. Your blood is pumping, your heart is pounding, and when you look down at your hands you see that they are clenched. Your teeth grind. Your eyes hurt. As it goes on longer and longer and your body stays ready for action, the bodily changes begin to take their toll. This is bad stress. If it continues, it is chronic. And that is very bad.

You see, when there is chronic stress, the problem is that the body does not slow itself back down. Instead of raising the blood pressure temporarily, chronic stress elevates blood pressure and leaves it up. In addition, pulse rate stays up.

What does this do? Well, it does a lot of detrimental things. It can lead to some serious illnesses. There are a number of conditions that appear to be related to chronic stress. These include some cases of diabetes, some heart conditions, some cases of high blood pressure, some stomach ulcers, some psychological changes, some forms of arthritis, some skin rashes, and certainly some headaches. Chronic stress may cause and will certainly aggravate all of these conditions. But worst of all, chronic stress aggravates chronic pain.

Stress Control

Due to chronic stress' unhealthy nature and profound effect on pain, it is essential that you take steps to recognize its causes. You need to manage and thus calm your stress. This is not as hard as you may think. But it's probably more important than you realize.

Consider the case of Fred, a quiet gentleman in his forties, who has facet disease. This is a derangement of one or more of the small joints in the spine that make bending and twisting possible. While visiting me, he said something that is probably familiar to almost anyone experiencing chronic pain.

"Tension makes it worse," said Fred. "In fact, tension can bring the pain on."

And so, what can be done?

Well, the first thing is to avoid or at least reduce stress chemicals, including: caffeine, salt, alcohol, and sugar. The next thing, and this may be a bit more difficult, is to do your best to avoid stressful situations. How?

:60 Second Stress Avoidance Advice

1. Arrive early for appointments. This is always less stressful than being just on time or late.
2. Allow extra time for travel since speeding, by itself, is stressful.
3. Try to get things done as early as possible instead of at the last minute.

You may notice that these three suggestions all have a similar theme—don't be rushing to catch up. When you rush, you place yourself in a stressful situation.

Here are some more suggestions:

---

4.   Have one *good* laugh a day. There really is something to the old saying, "Laughter is the best medicine." Not only does it make you happy, but it causes good chemical changes in your body.

5.   Do some exercise. Again, the chemical changes produced are good for you and exercise makes you feel stronger and more confident.

6.   Smile. Just like laughter, a smile produces chemical changes that go a long way toward reducing stress. Remember, your attitude is of the utmost importance.

7.   Do something creative. There are therapeutic activities out there that help in reducing stress. Among the best activities are those that exercise the creative side of your personality, including: art, music, crafts, poetry, and needlework.

8.   Remember your spiritual side. A spiritual belief of any kind is very helpful in reducing stress. A quiet conversation with God can help put your mind at ease.

You may notice that these suggestions also have a similar theme--your attitude *is* important so work on it.

Relaxation Response

You can do more than just avoiding stressful situations to reduce stress. In fact, there are proven exercises that not only calm the body but also calm the pain.

The exercises are not hard to learn.

The first is called Relaxation Response, which comes to us from Dr. Herbert Benson, Professor at Harvard Medical School and Deaconess Hospital in Boston. Relaxation Response, if done regularly, can lower your blood pressure, steady your pulse, and contribute to your general well-being in many ways.

:60 Second Exercises

The instructions go like this:

Find a comfortable chair in a quiet room. Take a seat and start to breathe, slowly and deeply.

As you breathe, concentrate on where those breaths come from, and try to bring the air deeply into your abdomen. You want this to be abdominal breathing. Slowly, deeply.

You want your diaphragm to push down, therefore pushing your abdomen out. Of course, your chest will expand too but concentrate on your abdomen. Nice and slow. Deep and slow. Steady. Steady.

When your breathing pattern is reasonably established, relax your hands and wrists. Think these words as you do: RELAX AND LET GO.

Slowly, deeply. RELAX AND LET GO. Feel the tension fall from your hands and wrists with each exhalation. RELAX AND LET GO. Feel it roll away.

Next, move to the muscles of your forearms. RELAX AND LET GO. Feel the tension as it releases from that specific part of your body. Easy, slow, deep. Breathe and relax.

Move on to your shoulder muscles. RELAX AND LET GO. Breathe and feel the stress wash away.

Continue on through other muscle groups: feet, ankles, calves, thighs, lower back, upper back, abdomen, chest, neck, face, and forehead. Just RELAX AND LET GO.

When you do this exercise, a number of things happen. By relaxing large muscles, the muscle fibers become loose and leave more room for blood to flow between them. The blood in a relaxed muscle washes away fatigue acids and other pain-producing chemicals. As the blood flow increases, you may experience a calm, pleasant feeling of warmth in the muscle that you relaxed. When you do so, you know you are having success in relaxing that muscle.

As you work your way up your body with the Relaxation Response exercise, you will begin to feel a calm come over you. Continue on from your forehead to your scalp, while breathing steady and slow, and with each breath you will feel the tension drain from your body.

After you have calmed yourself to a steady slow rhythm, concentrate on your area of pain and do the same exercise on that specific area. RELAX AND LET GO.

The wonderful thing about Relaxation Response is that it is a progressive exercise, meaning it becomes more helpful with each repetition. Make this exercise part of your daily routine.

Ideally, you should do this exercise in twenty minute intervals, twice a day. If you cannot sit still for an extended period like this, there is another way that is just as effective—do the Relaxation Response for three minutes at a time but once an hour. Think of these three minutes as your relaxation vacation. You will be amazed at the calming effect this has, not only on your pain, but also on your life.

Progressive Relaxation

Progressive Relaxation is another relaxation method you can use. It has been described by Dr. Edmund Jacobson, director of the Laboratory for Clinical Psychology in Chicago, as a combination of isometric exercises and relaxation response.

With this method, you tighten up a certain muscle before relaxing it. The reason for this is so that you can concentrate more fully on the muscle that you are relaxing.

The instructions go like this:

Sit in a comfortable chair in a quiet room. As you sit, concentrate on slow breaths and begin to search out different muscle groups. Begin with your hands.

Tighten your fists as hard as you can for ten seconds. If ten seconds is too long, start with less and gradually build up to it.

When the ten seconds are up, let your hands go as limp as possible while at the same time thinking RELAX AND LET GO. Feel the tension drain from your hands.

Next, move to your forearms and tighten them as taut as possible for ten seconds. Again, loosen them as much as possible while thinking RELAX AND LET GO.

Progressive Relaxation follows the same strategy as Relaxation Response by going through all of your muscle groups. Tighten for ten seconds and then release, thinking RELAX AND LET GO.

Next, in turn, try this exercise with: your upper arms, shoulders, toes, calves, thighs, abdomen, chest, lower back, upper back, neck in front, neck in back, face, forehead, and scalp. Tighten, then RELAX AND LET GO. Feel the drain and the warmth.

When you have relaxed all of your muscles in rotation, check your body systematically to make sure everything is relaxed. Breathe slowly and quietly. In and out. Deep, soft, quiet.

Visual Imagery

Once you have mastered techniques of relaxation and deep breathing, you can move onto the technique of visual imagery. Here you imagine peaceful, wonderful scenery and it's calming effect on your body and soul.

Stay in that comfortable chair in the quiet room. Close your eyes and keep your breathing steady and slow. Relax all of your muscles.

:60 Second Visual Imagery

Quietly conjure up an image of a wonderful, peaceful place, your favorite place—an outdoor location of soft breezes. It can be a seashore, lake, forest glade, or even your own backyard. Make it your favorite place, even if you've never been there. This is like the childhood game of imagination, only more peaceful.

It is important to fill in details. Think, imagine. If you are near water, are there whitecaps or is it as smooth as glass? What do you hear? Birds? Boats? You can never have enough details, and as you fill them in, remember to keep breathing, slowly, softly. Go there and let your mind take you in. Feel the sun, listen as a group of children giggle and run on the other side of the lake. Details, yes, soft and wonderful details.

You are at peace.

This exercise can be done twenty minutes at a time twice a day, or three minutes at a time every hour for a relaxation vacation. Enjoy it. This is your time.

Visual imagery can take many forms and here is another example that you can use specifically on your pain.

The instructions are:

Once you have relaxed, slowed, and steadied your breathing, begin to focus on your pain. Imagine you are marking the area of your pain with a pen. You are circling the area of your pain so that nothing outside that circle is in any pain. Now imagine that the circle of pain gets just a little smaller. The circle is slowly shrinking, smaller and smaller. Just a little. Breathe and shrink the circle. Progressively, you continue to shrink the circle.

Keep that pain in a smaller area but begin to shrink the intensity, just a little. Soften the pain. Change its definition. Breath by breath, feel the pain reduce itself to merely an ache.

Don't lie to yourself by trying to say the pain is all gone. That will get you nowhere. But shrink the pain in your imagination. Remember, the mind has immense powers.

There is another technique that is based on the experience of Eastern teachers of meditation: Go into a relaxed state again and this time use a mantra, or a one-word silent chant to yourself. You can use a word connected with your own religious experience or you can use a simple word, such as "peace," "success," "health," or "oneness." Concentrate on your breathing as you repeat that word over and over each time you exhale.

Visual imagery works exceptionally well, and there are many different ways to do it. A third way is to go back to imagining that lake or seashore. This time envision that there is a path between you and the water, and that you are walking along that path. Remember to think of details—what you are wearing and what you see along both sides of the path.

Keep walking and now imagine yourself with big happy strides. You swing your arms happily. Think of your face. It has a grin. Not just a small, upturned mouth, but an actual ear-to-ear grin. Why? Because you are happy!

Run with this thought. Feel the grin spread across your face. You are in a happy place, your favorite place in the whole world, and you are happy. Very happy. Let yourself revel in this happiness.

When you return to reality from your imagination, you will find yourself grinning still. Yes, this sounds simple, but it works. I know, I've tried it.

There is one more exercise to learn for visual imagery I want you to try. Go into complete relaxation again. This time, imagine a clear blue sky being crossed by a sky-writing airplane. As you look up, imagine you see the plane write "help!" across the sky in small letters.

As it does, imagine yourself whispering the word, *help!*

Now imagine the plane circling back and writing the word a bit bigger, *Help!*

And as it does, you imagine saying the word a bit louder, **HELP!**

And again, the plane comes back writing the word bigger still, and you say the word louder still.

Again the plane circles back. This time the plane writes the word HELP! so big that it covers the sky, and as it does, imagine yourself yelling at the top of your lungs, *Help!*

Now imagine one more thing.

Imagine that you are being heard!

Breathing Consciously

Breathing is an important tool in the battle for efficiency, relaxation, and pain control. As previously explained, diaphragmatic breathing at a steady pace is particularly important for pain control.

Pay close attention to the air you inhale and exhale. As you breathe in, feel the coolness of the air you inhale and as you breathe out, appreciate that what you exhale is much warmer. Sometimes, you'll taste moisture in the air and other times (perhaps in other places) you'll be aware of dryness in the air. Maybe you'll be cognizant of flowers, perfume, or even the sweet smell of bread baking. Enjoy it all. To breathe is to understand pleasure. Don't back away from it, but rather *revel* in it. Life is sweet, breathe it in.

When you do your relaxation exercises, pay attention to your respiration. This is not the only time you should take heed of what enters and leaves your lungs. Perhaps the best time to take notice of your respiration is when you exercise, because that is when you can feel "out of breath." However, if you approach exercise properly, you will learn to harness the power of proper breathing techniques.

For instance, when walking, consider counting two steps for inhalation and three or four steps for exhalation. The choice between three and four steps for exhalation is up to you and your level of physical fitness. The point is that you should have a system of breathing worked out before you begin exercising.

It is always wise to use more steps to exhale than to inhale. This way, you can empty your lungs more completely. You can also get rid of acids (among other things) more completely, as well as set yourself up for a quick and efficient inhalation.

You should work on this plan with a degree of flexibility, depending on your own level of physical conditioning. For instance, you could inhale every three steps versus exhaling for the next five or six steps. The same principle applies to running or climbing, but each individual should work out their own system since only they know their own capabilities.

Conscious breathing, no matter the exercise, increases efficiency. The point is that a conscious effort to control breathing takes your mind off negative thoughts. Remember, the mind has immense powers. Breathing is just one tool that can be used to tap into these powers.

Hypnosis

The antics of a stage hypnotist are well-known but have little medical relevance. Additionally, hypnosis, as seen in old movies with a swinging watch, has very little to do with hypnosis techniques used by those in the medical professions.

Hypnosis can be effective as a relaxation exercise if it is brought on by a trained professional. Patients can learn to self-hypnotize, and do not have to become dependent upon a hypnotist.

Most professionals start with relaxation routines. Hypnosis is much like Relaxation Response. The patient is taught to deepen the hypnotic state by various suggestions. One such method is to have the patient count backward from ten as instructions are given to relax. Each number brings about a happier, calmer, more relaxed state. When a patient reaches an optimum state of relaxation, he or she is ready to receive suggestions about pain relief.

The problem is the percentage of cases in which hypnosis is successful in alleviating chronic pain for long periods of time is quite low. Other stress control methods have a higher percentage of success. However, in some patients, the hypnosis method results in some pain control.

If you have tried other methods and still not found relief, trying hypnotism may be beneficial.

Insomnia

Anyone who suffers from chronic pain knows how desperately important it is to get sleep. You know, in fact, that good sleep is a great blessing. If you have had a restful night's sleep, you probably had an easier time dealing with the pain. However, worrying about whether you will sleep well will only make the situation worse, and also tends to make sleeping more difficult.

It is probably wise to accept whatever quirks nature has wished on us in the matter of sleep. The number of hours of sleep needed varies from person to person. For each individual, it may even change from day to day or week to week. As a rule, you generally get as much sleep as you need, however if you are in chronic pain, you may not. If you worry about it constantly, you will find yourself undergoing stress. You have learned previously how bad stress can complicate your chronic pain. It can seem like a vicious circle; you are in pain because you can't sleep, and you can't sleep because you are in pain.

There are a number of things other than pills that may help. (Of course, if your doctor prescribes a pill, it is all right to take it.)

:60 Second Sleep Advice

1.   Make sure you have a combination of physical and mental activities throughout the day. If you have spent your whole day sitting on a couch, don't expect to fall asleep easily when you go to bed. If you are not tired physically, it is difficult to fall asleep. Simple. Therefore, you need to get at least a moderate amount of physical exercise every day. You don't need to run a marathon or do anything strenuous which will exhaust you, but you do want enough exercise to feel a slight ache in your muscles. You also want to have a degree of mental exhaustion. Reading, watching television or listening to soothing music may help. You want to get into bed with the feeling that you have used both your body and your mind throughout the day.

2.   If you have a pre-sleep routine that has worked for you before, use it. Even if your method is counting sheep, use it. If you believe in hot milk before bed, drink it. A snack is helpful for some, while prayerful meditations are helpful for others.

3.   Your stomach should not be too full or too empty. Every individual is different. Try several eating techniques to find out what is right for you.

4.   Have a notebook and pen at your bedside. It is common to remember things that must be done just when you would like to empty your mind and go to sleep. When this happens, write the item in your notebook and assign yourself a definite time and date

when you will do it. Once you've written the assignment down, stop worrying about it. You have it noted down and don't need to keep it in mind, prohibiting you from relaxing and drifting into sleep.

5. Ask yourself, "What did I enjoy today? Did I see, hear, or read anything interesting?" If you dwell on a happy event, inevitably it will promote sleep. If nothing pleasant happened today, tell yourself, "Tomorrow will be better because I want it to be better."

6. Do your relaxation exercises and visual imagery exercises using images of sleep.

7. Keep track of your use of caffeine. The cut-off time for regular coffee is different for each individual, although a general rule of no caffeine after noon may be helpful to you.

8. Do not use alcohol as a sleeping medicine. Alcohol induced sleep is *not* healthy sleep.

9. Try reading before you go to sleep, but select your reading material carefully. Right before bedtime is not the best time to read a thriller. Instead, try reading something peaceful or meditative.

10. Try listening to gentle music.

The best advice for getting a restful night's sleep is to be flexible until you find something that works. When you find a combination that works, make it part of your routine.

Stress and Sleep

You can promote a more restful night of sleep, thus helping reduce stress, with an individual routine. Don't give up and don't get frustrated. There will always be some level of stress in your life. However, the important thing is to recognize it and take control of it. With practice, you can learn to get into your relaxation mode in less than :60 seconds.

Chapter 5

Controlling Problem Habits

Generally, things we do routinely that make our life happier, more effective, and more of a joy to others are defined as good habits. These habits are sustained by an optimism about the future.

There are a number of habits that are counterproductive in the battle against pain and they are most often grounded in a profound pessimism about the outcome of chronic pain.

List your bad health habits:

:60 Second Bad Habits List

1.   PESSIMISM—negative thought pattern
2.   CAFFEINE—increases your awareness of pain
3.   TOBACCO—health risk
4.   OVEREATING—excess weight can increase pain
5.   OVERUSE OF NARCOTICS—threat to independence, health and emotional well being
6.   ABUSE OF ALCOHOL—physical, emotional dangers

Let's look at these one at a time:

Pessimism

Pessimism comes from the Latin word, "pessimus," meaning: the worst. It indicates the tendency to look for the worst possibilities in every situation. For a person in chronic pain, it is very easy and also very destructive to look for the worst possibilities.

The damage is not only psychological, but I believe that it also inhibits the production of chemicals in the body that help us to be active and fight pain.

A negative thought pattern is a bad habit. And with proper care, it can be kicked.

How do you recognize pessimism? With very little imagination, you can think of fifty possibilities that are positive or negative. Your thoughts are usually a mixture of both, but pay attention to the direction your thinking takes.

:60 Second Definition (Pessimist)

Here is a good example of a pessimist: one who has a headache and believes it is a brain tumor. Such negative foreshadowing of future possibilities is known to behavioral scientists as "awfulizing." Of course, there is not a shred of reality to this pessimism in most cases. The time utilized in this pessimistic thinking is an avoidable waste.

If you have nothing good to say about your own situation, soon you will have nothing good to say about anything or anybody else. You may also realize that you don't have anything good to say about yourself. That is dangerous, as you must treat yourself with respect.

Pessimism often has no basis in reality. The only way to get rid of pessimism is to replace it with a good thought pattern habit—optimism.

So what is and how do you get optimism? First off, understand that optimism also comes from a Latin word, "optimus," meaning the best. You can't get optimism from pills or shots. It doesn't work that way. Optimism can only come from inside yourself. It comes from a driven determination to look on the bright side of things. Obviously, you cannot do this on command. Like all good things in life, you have to work at it.

:60 Second Ways to Work Toward Optimism

1.　　When you read a book, make an effort to stop at an upbeat word or upbeat sentence. The thought process that this will trigger can have a profound effect on the next hour of your life.

2.　　Listen to cheerful music (music that makes you happy or that you associate with a happy moment in your life).

3.　　Praise yourself. You deserve it.

4.　　Remember things you have accomplished and remind yourself that you can do it again.

5.　　When you see something beautiful, such as a sunset, sunrise, flower, picture, or whatever moves you, share it with someone. Draw their attention to it. Just talking about beautiful scenes will improve your outlook.

6.　　Think of happy moments from your life.

7.　　Play pretend games of optimism even when you are not in the mood. Pretend you are interested in beauty. Pretend that beautiful music pleases you. You just may find yourself getting caught up in this game of pretend.

Caffeine

Caffeine is the active substance in coffee, tea, cola, and cocoa. It is very enjoyable when used sparingly; but it is habit forming in many cases. Caffeine can also reinforce pain in some chronic pain sufferers.

One thing is certain, caffeine narrows the small blood vessels which can cause a rise in blood pressure. This can be dangerous if you have a problem with circulation. It can also cause or aggravate irregular heartbeat in some people.

Caffeine makes you more alert and aware. Obviously this is good if you want to do some difficult reading or studying, but it will also make you more aware of your pain.

In fact, caffeine can have such an adverse effect that it can actually counteract some of the medicines that are prescribed to relieve pain.

:60 Second Caffeine Quiz

Do you use caffeine (coffee, tea, etc.)?	Yes	No
Does it affect you?	Yes	No
Does it cause:		
Headaches	Yes	No
Fast heartbeat	Yes	No
Irregular heartbeat	Yes	No
Nervousness	Yes	No
Higher blood pressure	Yes	No
Hunger	Yes	No
Heartburn or stomach ache	Yes	No
Irritability	Yes	No
Insomnia	Yes	No
Has your doctor asked you to cut or quit your intake?	Yes	No

If you answered yes to two questions, it is advisable to stop ingesting caffeine. Three yes answers makes it urgent to abstain from this substance. And, obviously, if you answered yes to the last question, you really have no choice.

Clearly, it is best to cut down or, if possible, eliminate the use of caffeine. But how?

Some people have managed to stop all at once, what is referred to as "cold turkey." This is not easy, and attempts can often be unsuccessful and therefore frustrating, leading to another bad habit—pessimism.

Here is one suggestion: cut your intake of regular coffee, tea, cola, or whatever you drink by one cup a week. For instance, if you normally drink ten cups of coffee a day, cut down to nine cups of regular coffee and one cup of decaffeinated. Stick with this for a week. The next week, cut to eight cups of regular coffee and two cups of decaf. It makes the transition easier. Continue this week by week until you are down to zero caffeinated drinks.

Robert's Caffeine Story

Robert is in his early forties. He is a slender, high-strung and intense man who works for a large computer company. Robert's problem is quite common at that company; he suffers from headaches. At first, it seemed that his problems were directly related to stress on the job. However, in discussing Robert's problem and a typical day with him, I discovered another potential cause of tension headaches.

Robert drank fifteen cups of black coffee everyday as he went about his stressful duties. Now certainly, short of quitting, his duties were not going to disappear, nor were they destined to become less stressful. Business, after all, is business. I theorized that all that caffeine in his coffee was at the very least aggravating the problem. When Robert finally realized his intake was adversely affecting his health and productivity on the job, he heroically quit cold turkey. His headaches almost disappeared.

Smoking

You know smoking is bad for you. You cannot have been around for the past twenty or thirty years and not realize its devastating effects. However, did you know that in addition to the overall health problems smoking causes, it also has an effect on chronic pain?

Whenever there is a disturbance in the function of the blood vessels, smoking can aggravate the condition considerably, sometimes resulting in chronic pain.

When blood vessels are open reasonably wide, blood can wash out fatigue, stress, and pain chemicals. But nicotine narrows blood vessels, which makes some pains worse.

It is absolutely beneficial to quit smoking. The good news is, there are effective ways to quit smoking.

Here are six steps to stop smoking:

1) Smoke every hour (on the hour). Smoke one cigarette or less, but never more. If you skip an hour for any reason, do not try to catch up. Smoke the next hour. The idea is to get some control over your smoking. This routine should continue for a few months. Make it a habit. The length of time to continue step 1 should be proportionate to the amount you smoke. A one-pack-a-day smoker should stay with this for two to three months. A two-pack-a-day smoker should stay with this three to five months. Once you have control over the one hour pattern, move on.

2) Smoke one cigarette every two hours. This step should also be continued for two to five months, until you have control over this pattern. If at some point you don't feel the need to finish the cigarette, don't. Then you will be ready for the next step.

3) Smoke one cigarette every four hours. Continue this for one month.

4) Smoke one cigarette three times a day. Continue this for one month.

5) Smoke one cigarette twice a day. Again, continue until you have control over this pattern.

6) You are now ready to quit. Good luck! Do relapses occur? Maybe. If they do, don't despair. Just return to the step at which you were when the relapse occurred.

:60 Second Smokefree Reminders

•Control is a skill that must be practiced. The gradual, paced program you have read is ideal for this purpose.

•General health comes first. It is pointless to work on pain and neglect your general health. By quitting smoking, you will improve your general health.

•Some pains are aggravated by smoking. In these cases, smoking works against your purpose: pain control.

Overweight

Excess pounds can be burdensome for a person in chronic pain, especially if the pain is in the lower part of the body. The extra pressure put on the body is not healthy. Most likely, it adds more pain.

There is a joke that describes such a situation:

If you are too heavy for your height, you have two choices. You can grow a few inches, or lose the weight. Do whichever one is easier.

Truthfully, though, weight control is especially beneficial for someone experiencing chronic pain. Excess weight tends to make people less inclined to be active. Moreover, controlling weight is a great morale builder, and good morale is essential in your fight to diminish pain.

If you find yourself in need of weight loss, it is important to approach a diet with the proper attitude.

Don't expect miracles. Instead, you should set reasonable goals.

:60 Second Weight Loss Suggestions

First, consult your doctor. Your choice of weight loss methods should be guided by your doctor's advice about your general health, condition, and needs. Your doctor knows best.

Second, keep a food diary listing all that you eat for a week. Show this to your doctor.

Third, set a goal. A goal of losing one pound a week is not unreasonable. Crash diets don't usually work because the rebound effect can bring all the weight back as fast as you lost it. Instead, approach weight loss with a controlled attitude.

This slow weight-loss schedule will enable you to establish good eating and living habits so you can maintain the proper weight once your goal has been reached. In fact, if you begin losing weight, you are likely to experience some pain relief long before you have reached your ideal weight.

This is not a diet book and I will not list the many kinds of diets that work. However, I will give some general points and suggest one diet which I've found effective. Eat a varied diet, and you'll be safe whether you take vitamin pills or not.

Green and yellow vegetables and fruits are a very important source of nutrition. Pasta, potatoes, and whole grain bread are also part of a good diet. Try to concentrate on starches, not sugars, and avoid all unnecessary fat. Remove fat from meat before it is cooked or it will cook into the meat. Be sure you eat the foods you are supposed to eat. Try and stick with things which are good for you and are permitted on your individual diet plan. Salads are good for roughage, and complex carbohydrates, such as potatoes, noodles, whole grain breads, or cereals are good "energy foods." As for cooking, it is much healthier to boil, bake, or broil that it is to fry.

Fourth, never skip a meal and then gorge later. In fact, you may be better off eating more meals of smaller portions than you are eating three larger meals a day. Make a schedule and then stick with it.

Fifth, keep track of your inner feelings. If you are feeling full, or no longer hungry, it is a good sign that you should stop eating. In three or four hours, you will be eating another meal.

:60 Second Suggested Weight Reduction Diet

If you are going to try this diet, remember to consult your physician.

Start with a light breakfast each day. Go easy on the eggs, only having one egg occasionally. Instead, try whole grain cereal, low-fat or no-fat milk, juice, and citrus fruit.

Between breakfast and lunch, have a light snack.

I recommend some whole wheat crackers or broth, and some decaffeinated tea or coffee.

There are many possibilities for lunch, but stay within your diet. Some possibilities include whole grain bread, low-fat cottage cheese, salad with oil and vinegar or a fat-free dressing, fruit, or whole grain cereal with low-fat, or no-fat milk. For a drink, perhaps some herbal tea or decaffeinated tea or coffee.

Between lunch and dinner, have another small snack—perhaps fruit or low-fat cottage cheese and a couple of crackers.

Most people want to consume meat for dinner. If this is the case, it is best to stick with chicken, fish, or veal. A small to medium baked potato is also good for some people. (Again, check with your physician.) Two green vegetables and one yellow one should be part of this meal. Meat should be baked, broiled, or, if suitable, boiled. Chicken skin and meat fat should be removed *before* cooking.

If you get hungry after dinner, you may have a tiny snack. However, in order to have a late night snack, you have to save up sufficient unconsumed calories from the day. Your snack should fit into your overall caloric scheme. Some possibilities include: fruit juice, clear broth, high-grain crackers, and fat-free milk.

You may wonder how you can lose weight with the six meal menu I've described. Actually, you're taking the food you would normally be consuming on your diet and redistributing it into five or six meals. It

works. I have found that people on a multiple meal program have an easier time losing weight than those who
stick to three meals a day.

Don't worry too much about relapses. They are
natural. Once you have one, don't turn it into a major
drama, that can result in a pessimistic attitude. Instead,
resolve to get back onto your program.

Remember to pay attention to the feeling of
being full or not being hungry. Once you are able to
recognize these feelings, you will find that they come a
little sooner during the meal. That may indicate your
stomach has gotten a bit smaller. This is progress! You
are gaining control!

:60 Second Weight Loss Tips

---

1.   Every day, write down everything you eat
or drink, the amount, and the calories. You will need a
caloric table for this.

2.   Weigh yourself every morning. Do it
without any clothes on.

3.   Try to correlate the food diary with what
you learn from your scale. Soon, you will know the
number of calories you need to maintain your weight. You
will also know how many calories will cause a weight
gain, and how many will bring a weight loss.

The important principle behind the :60 Second
Suggested Diet and the :60 Second Weight Loss tips is

that they make you conscious of everything you eat. This is essential when you are trying for slow, steady weight loss. It is a flexible program as well that gives you a certain number of freedoms. If you take in some extra calories at one meal (such excesses will happen from time to time), just cut down on the next two meals. This way, you control not just your weight but also your food intake.

:60 Second Weight Control Summary

---

1.   Your general health comes first.
2.   If the pain is in the lower half of your body, extra pounds can add to your suffering.
3.   Learning control is essential.
4.   Weight control will build up your morale, and a good attitude is your best weapon against chronic pain.

Overuse of Narcotics

Narcotics are useful medicines. They are very powerful, but they can also bring on severe complications and side effects.

In the right cases, narcotics may act as agents to relieve pain. For instance, narcotics have been found to be quite helpful for cancer patients experiencing severe pain.

Narcotics are also called opioids. Many come

from natural sources such as the poppy plant grown in Asia. In the last few years, some have been manufactured synthetically.

These medicines act on the surface of cells, particularly on nerve cells. The areas in which they work are called Opioid Receptors. (As was pointed out earlier, this is the same area where the body's natural pain fighters, endorphins, work.)

Narcotics are good pain relievers for acute, severe pain. They are particularly useful if used for a short time. This limited usage avoids some of the more serious complications, such as addictions.

For practical purposes, we can divide narcotics into three groups:

1. Mild Narcotics—such as Codeine
2. Strong Narcotics—such as Morphine or Demerol
3. Long-Lasting Narcotics—such as Methadone

Mild narcotics are frequently used for pain in such injuries as fractures, and are often taken by prescription at home. Strong narcotics are beneficial in fighting pain after operations. Long-lasting narcotics have been used in weaning addicted patients from their drug of choice. In order to alleviate discomfort and severe pain, long-lasting narcotics are also used to treat cancer patients.

In the case of chronic pain, many pain specialists

generally prefer to avoid prescribing narcotics. They believe, and I also am among those who have this opinion, that too many complications can occur.

:60 Second Narcotics Complication Information

1.   In the course of time, the same dose of the same drug will have a decreased effect on the pain; so the interval between needed doses becomes shorter. This is called tolerance.

2.   Physical dependence may happen if a medicine is taken for a period of time, even a short period of time. The body may then respond violently if the medicine is taken away. This abstinence syndrome is colloquially known as cold turkey. When a person quits taking a substance on which they are physically dependent, they can develop several symptoms. For instance, they can develop chills and gooseflesh at the slightest draft of air. However, there are more potential problems than mere gooseflesh. A person going through withdrawal often develops pain and cramps from digestive activity, and any normal touch or activity can also be excruciatingly painful. To lessen these symptoms, drugs must be tapered off gradually. It is also important to remember that long-term use of narcotics blocks the production of endorphins.

3.   Psychological dependence on a sub-

stance is also known as addiction. People who are addicted become obsessed with the idea that he/she must have the drug and will stop at nothing to get it. In cases like this, it is common for a physician to hear things like, "I lost the bottle," or "The dog ate my pills," or "I dropped them into the sink." An addicted individual who can't get a particular substance may try to falsify prescriptions, get prescriptions from a number of physicians, or even buy or trade for narcotics in the black market.

List the medications you take:

:60 Second Addiction Symptoms

1.	Constipation
2.	Nausea
3.	Sedation, sleepiness
4.	Lightheadedness
5.	Respiratory Depression in which breathing becomes less frequent. In cases of severe overdose, breathing may stop entirely.
6.	Euphoria or Dysphoria. Euphoria is an overly happy feeling without legitimate reason. This is dangerous because it can lead to psychological addiction. Dysphoria is a deep unhappiness without legitimate reason. This also can lead to addictions.
7.	Dry Mouth
8.	Muscle Rigidity
9.	Urinary Retention, difficulty to pass urine
10.	Itchiness

If a dangerous habit results from intake, it is often necessary to use hospital treatment for safe withdrawal, as well as prolonged psychological or psychiatric care. Withdrawal may be too much for a person to handle on his or her own. Remember, to consider the aforementioned consequences before you take prescribed narcotics. Make this a responsible decision arrived at with your physician. Above all, never take drugs prescribed for someone else.

Alcohol Abuse

There is evidence that a small amount of alcohol intake may be good for some people. That evidence may or may not hold up to further scrutiny.

However, there is no doubt that a daily intake of a large amount of alcohol is unhealthy for both the body and the mind. Unquestionably, alcohol *abuse* is bad.

Alcohol is especially harmful for someone experiencing chronic pain. For one thing, it interferes with the body's production of substances to fight pain. It also has a punishing effect on the liver and other organs.

In addition, alcohol, especially beer, adds useless calories to your diet. This is bad for those chronic pain sufferers who are overweight, and for those with pain in the lower part of the body.

There is a myth to be cleared up about alcohol. It has been said often, and erroneously, that when a person has had too much to drink that person is "feeling no pain." According to this perception, everything else is dulled and judgment has become clouded.

Actually, imbibing large amounts of alcohol creates future pain. The intoxicated person may be engaging in self-destructive override at night. But by morning, many of the body's natural chemicals used to fight pain have been used to fight the ravages of alcohol. Alcohol, like some narcotics, interferes with the production of endorphins, and also with the long-

term functioning of the immune system. The body
can end up less able to fight pain, stress, infection, or
even cancer.

If you wonder whether you have an alcohol
problem, you probably do. Please seek advice. It is a
dangerous habit.

There are many types of alcoholics: the weekend
drinker, the binge drinker, and the person who craves
the first drink of the day earlier and begins making
drinks larger.

Many have recognized their problem and have
quit. Some were able to quit by themselves, others cannot do it alone. They must seek help, they need medical
advice, and sometimes it is necessary for them to enter
a rehabilitation hospital.

The fight against alcohol dependency can be a
lonely fight; therefore, it can be useful to join a program
such as Alcoholics Anonymous. Some religious organi-
zations also run good rehabilitation programs.

If you drink to excess, you are not giving your body
or your mind a fair chance in your fight against pain.

Chapter 6

Special Pain Conditions

Chronic pain comes in many different forms, and sometimes behaves strangely. Some forms are more insidious than others. Some are more difficult to explain, and some require different treatments. Often a mixture of acute and chronic pain is present that can be confusing and irksome.

If you are able to face your pain condition with knowledge, you will be more equipped for the battle to diminish it.

List your pain symptoms:

:60 Second Special Pain Conditions Survey

---

1.   Sympathetic Dystrophy
2.   Peripheral Neuralgia
3.   Post-Herpetic Neuralgia
4.   Osteoporosis
5.   Fibromyalgia
6.   Amputation Pain
    A.   Stump Pain
    B.   Phantom Pain
7.   Torticollis (Wry Neck)
8.   Cancer Pain

In all of these conditions you need good medical advice, and sometimes surgical or other treatment. Your participation in the process will insure its success.

Sympathetic Dystrophy

The human body has two nervous systems.

One is called the somatic system. This system encompasses all the nerves that have to do with sensation—feeling, touch, the sense organs, warmth, cold, pain, and motion.

The other system is called the autonomic nervous system, which works very well without our conscious influence. This system controls, among other things, heart rate, breathing and the functions of the bowels, stomach, and bladder.

The autonomic nervous system is further divided into the sympathetic nervous system and the parasympathetic nervous system, which are mirror images of each other.

For instance, the sympathetic nervous system can speed up the heart rate while the parasympathetic nervous system can slow it down. When you are healthy, these two systems are in balance.

These two systems also control blood pressure by narrowing or relaxing smaller arteries in the periphery of the body. This is very useful in the case of danger. When there is an emergency, blood vessels in the skin automatically narrow and thus, blood is shuttled to the muscles, heart, and brain as needed.

This is a very effective and efficient system, when it works well. It is not when it performs an emergency function without an emergency. (See Chapter 4.)

When a large somatic nerve is disrupted, especially if it is only partially cut, some of its function is lost. If this happens, the sympathetic nerves will *attempt* to take over. I say "attempt" because they are not very successful.

In trying to make up for the function of destroyed nerves, the sympathetic nerves tend to narrow blood vessels too much. This condition is called sympathetic dystrophy.

It was discovered by a perceptive physician, Dr. Weir Mitchell, during the American Civil War. Dr.

Mitchell called the condition "causalgia," meaning burning pain. This is an appropriate description of what a patient feels.

If the blood vessels narrow, not enough blood goes to the extremities—the hand, foot, or some other part of the body. When this happens, the extremity involved (most commonly a hand or foot) becomes cold. It also turns pale or blue and is extremely sensitive to touch. Considerable damage can be caused to blood vessels, muscles, nerves, or even bones. If the condition persists, it can do permanent damage.

Fortunately, we can stop the activity of the sympathetic nerves by injecting a local anesthetic into the ganglion, the life center of the nerve. The nerve, in effect, is put to sleep temporarily and releases blood vessels into the area affected. Thereafter, the part affected becomes warm and free of pain. The effect is quite startling, but the injections must be repeated.

Over time, the intervals between repeat injections become longer. This indicates that the sympathetic nerves have become less overactive. There are also some drugs that can be taken orally that have a similar effect.

Another way to combat the sensation of cold is to use certain Relaxation Response techniques combined with visual imagery. You can actually reproduce the effect of the injection with your imagination (see Chapter 4). Remember, the mind is stronger than the body.

Consider the story of Ella.

Ella, who is in her late thirties, had been hurt in a work accident in which her hand was caught in a roller and severely damaged. She came into my office cradling her left hand in a pillow that she was carrying in her right hand. She was suffering from sympathetic dystrophy of the left hand. The hand was a pale blue and extremely cold because the arteries in that part of her body had narrowed and almost completely shut down.

We tried injections, and Ella reacted quite well. The injection caused an immediate warming of her hand. The hand became pink and a great deal less painful.

However, Ella did not want to have continuous injections. She was not a fan of needles. No one is. So I worked with Ella, teaching her relaxation techniques that helped circulation and allowed her to avoid the numerous injections.

We also worked on some visual imagery techniques. I told her to imagine she was dipping her hand into a barrelful of hot water and steam was rising from the hand. These techniques seemed to work for her.

One day, she came to the office for a necessary injection because her hand had become discolored and cold. However, because injections cause some numbness, I insist that all patients receiving an injection have someone else drive them home from such appointments.

On this particular day, Ella came without a driver. I insisted that I would not give the shot until she had a driver.

"I'll be back," she said.

She returned as promised. But when I examined her again, her hand was pink and warm. It was an incredible change in just a few hours. I was so astonished I asked, "What happened?"

"I just did the exercises that you taught me," she said with a smile.

For the most part, Ella was able to keep herself from having too much pain. She had become very skilled at mental manipulation.

Peripheral Neuralgia

Neuralgia means pain in a nerve—usually in an extremity or the shoulders, neck, scalp, or face.

There can be many causes of this condition including: diabetes, alcohol abuse, heavy metal poisoning and the pain following an attack of shingles (which will be discussed later in greater detail).

The pain is often described as nagging, numb, burning, dull, and sharp. Different descriptions can all adequately define this type of pain. Whatever description fits, this type of pain is a special challenge.

The most important factor is a clear diagnosis. This involves a thorough neurological examination, often including an electro-myogram. An electro-myogram is a test in which muscles and nerves are stimulated by a weak electric current. The muscles reaction to the current is then measured.

Once there is a diagnosis, we study the underlying

cause. If the cause can be corrected, this is a priority. For example, diabetes must be fully controlled before there is any hope of pain control in diabetic neuritis. Unfortunately, there are no guarantees of success. The only guarantee is that the patient definitely will not get better until the underlying cause is controlled.

A number of measures are useful in treating peripheral neuralgia. For example vitamins, especially the B complex group, are frequently ordered. In many cases, the application of pepper extract ointments (Zostrix, or the generic form, Capsaicin) are successful. TENS machines, which provide electric stimulation, are less successful but worth trying. Non-steroidal anti-inflammatory drugs (aspirin, ibuprofen, and others) also work well in some cases.

Sometimes neuralgia (nerve pain) is experienced along with neuritis (nerve inflammation). It can be helpful to stabilize the surface layers of nerve fibers to reduce the speed of electrical and chemical changes in the nerve. This can control the transmission of pain signals. Anti-convulsant drugs such as Dilantin or Tegretol can also do this in some patients. When you combine the drugs with anti-depressants such as amitriptyline (Elavil), there can be a soothing influence on pain nerves.

Another treatment method that is frequently successful is the intravenous injection of a dilute solution of Lidocaine, a local anesthetic with a proven ability to stabilize the heartbeat. It has a similar influence on neuritis and neuralgia.

In the case of alcoholic neuritis, if the patient quits drinking, it will not always stop the condition. However, continued pain will result if the patient doesn't stop drinking.

None of these medications or treatments work for all people, but they work well for some.

But the biggest adjustment the patient has to make is with his or her own attitude. If you become depressed, no one should blame you; but remember, depression is counterproductive. Actually, as I've said elsewhere in this book, depression reduces the pain-fighting chemicals in your body.

It is essential to pay attention to mood, stress habits, and other problems. Nothing is marginal. Your mood is a weapon in your battle against pain.

Either use it or fall victim to it.

If you use it, you will win.

Post-Herpetic Neuralgia

About 10 percent of all people who get shingles end up with post-herpetic neuralgia which can cause chronic pain. Generally post-herpetic neuralgia affects older people.

What is shingles? It is a painful disease caused by the same virus that infects people with chickenpox. When childhood or adult chickenpox disappears, it does not go away. It stays in the body, usually near one of the nerve centers, which are called ganglia.

For an unknown reason, in some people the virus later becomes active. When it does, it attacks the ganglion, the nerve root, or other parts of the nervous system. The pain can be in just one nerve. Often it is under one rib, but it can also involve neighboring nerves. For example, three or four ribs may be affected. Sometimes pain is on one side of the face or part of a leg. It is a strong pain, like an acute pain. However, the discussion of treatment for shingles is for another forum.

Once the shingles are gone after effective treatment, some people develop post-herpetic neuralgia—a chronic nerve pain. This pain usually occurs in the same area as the attack of shingles. The pain can be quite severe. It can be a burning or a burning and numbness. Some have described the pain as a feeling of ants crawling on the skin. There is a constant ache in the painful area and a feeling of weakness.

Patients sometimes have an accompanying depression. The depression can snowball and cause the patient to neglect eating and drinking liquids. This can cause other health problems. As in all depression cases, they should be treated as soon as possible. A patient who is depressed and prescribed anti-depressants may benefit because some of these drugs are effective in reducing pain as well as reducing depression. Other types of medications used along with electrical stimulation, injections, ointments, etc. may also be used.

Post-herpetic neuralgia is a complicated disease. It must be attacked from many sides, experimenting with many different types of treatment. For example, one treatment that sometimes works is an injection of a mixture of local anesthetics and steroids into the painful area. If detection is early, sympathetic or other nerve blocks sometimes work. However, frequently patients with post-herpetic neuralgia are seen too late in the disease for these treatments to do much good. Medications such as Tylenol and Codeine can also work for a time, but they do not have a lasting effect. Some patients with post-herpetic neuralgia may benefit from Zostrix ointment. Remember:

•Nothing works for everyone.
•Everything is worth trying.
•But most important of all is
psychological management.

The mind is more powerful than the body. Once you understand that, you can begin to fight your pain on the most important level. If you develop a good attitude, your pain can be managed more easily.

Attitude. Don't let it bring you down. Remember the concept of *override*, as it works even for people with post-herpetic neuralgia. (See the section on override.)

Truthfully, the battle is never won. It is always being fought. The pain can be overcome for a while, but it returns and must be overcome again and again. You must make repeated psychological onslaughts on the condition. It is a take-no-prisoners, day-to-day effort.

I have seen many patients use this strategy and find success. I also have seen other people resigned to their pain. They had given up. They had made no effort to participate in their health care team.

In direct proportion, those who understand their roles as the most important member of their health care team will inevitably figure out a way to succeed.

Osteoporosis

Also known as brittle bone disease, osteoporosis is characterized by a progressive loss of bone tissues. The most frequent symptom is bone fractures. There are occasional cases where young people are affected, but usually this disease hits people over fifty.

The disease is actually a mixture of acute and chronic pain. When new fractures occur, they tend to be acutely painful. But in some cases a new fracture happens so often that it acquires many of the characteristics of chronic pain.

There are two types of osteoporosis. Type one osteoporosis affects more women than men by a ratio of 6-1. In women, it often follows menopause and is due, in great part, to a lack of hormones.

The most characteristic fractures for type one osteoporosis are those of the vertebrae and the wrist. Fractures of the vertebrae cause many patients to walk and stand with a bent or hunched back.

Type two osteoporosis affects people in old age.

Women are twice as likely as men to suffer from it. Fractures of the hip, vertebrae, shoulder, upper arm, and shinbone are common. This condition is probably caused by the inability of the aging body to absorb or utilize vitamin D properly.

This type of osteoporosis can be due to a hormone imbalance or to certain medications such as Cortisone. Other things such as alcohol, smoking, sleeping pills (barbituates), and Heparin (a drug to prevent blood clotting) may also bring on this condition.

The best treatment is prevention. For women, proper hormone treatment, if not contraindicated, appears to work well.

Regular exercise is another important preventative. Most people who come down with osteoporosis were not in the habit of exercising.

Treatments for those with the disease include the aforementioned hormones as well as back support garments, heat applications, and stretching exercises. Calcium supplements can help prevent bones from deteriorating further and may help build up bone tissue.

Fibromyalgia

This kind of pain affects muscles, tendons, and other connective tissue. The patient feels pain, stiffness, limitation of motion, weakness, and sometimes disturbances of blood flow to connected areas.

One characteristic symptom of fibromyalgia is

the appearance of trigger points. When you touch a patient at a trigger point, he or she will feel the pain, but not necessarily there. The pain may be felt at a different point on the body, perhaps on a trail from the trigger point up the course of a long muscle, tendon, or nerve.

To diagnose fibromyalgia, you look for a pain history of at least six months and at least six trigger points. There may even be up to eighteen trigger points. Another symptom is chronic fatigue, and yet another is depression. The depression, of course, should be treated first.

The best treatment is a global approach, meaning trying many different things. Trigger points are treated with injections. TENS machines often work well. I also recommend counseling, antidepressant drugs when necessary, and a gentle exercise program.

When there is energetic management using all of these different components, patients with fibromyalgia can improve. It may take time (sometimes months), but if the patient can stay positive, he or she can be helped.

Amputation Pain

Pain following an amputation can be very severe. There are two forms:

1.   Stump Pain.

This condition arises from the cut nerve or nerves in the amputated area. Sometimes the cut nerves grow into a knot-like formation called a neuroma. This

formation is sensitive to touch and makes the wearing
of a prosthesis very difficult. Surgery is sometimes
needed to remove the neuroma itself. In certain cases,
surgery on the spinal cord is necessary.

Local injections above the neuroma can be temporarily useful. Also, use of anti- depressant drugs such
as amitriptilynes have been helpful in some cases. I
have also seen a TENS machine be effective. However,
this machine cannot always be applied on the stump or
on the side with the pain. Application of electrodes to
the opposite side (the side not amputated) works in
many cases. The electronic message gets back to the
centers in the brain or spine and helps fight pain.

2.   Phantom Pain.

It is not unusual for post-amputation patients to
have phantom feelings in the amputated part (as if it
were still attached to the patient). The symptom can be
both puzzling and annoying. It is much worse if the sensation is one of pain. Phantom pain can be quite severe.

A number of treatments for this problem have
been tried with varying success. Some patients have had
success using a TENS machine. This machine sometimes provides relief when applied to the wrong side.

Standard pain medications such as narcotics or
non-steroidal anti-inflammatories are effective in some
cases. Sometimes injections are helpful, especially
spinal injections or injections into the epidural space.

Amputation is not just a physical trauma. It is a
severe psychological trauma as well. Therefore, it is

important to consider counseling, medication, and stress reduction. All could have an impact on your ability to deal with phantom pain.

One piece of knowledge may provide those who suffer from it a measure of consolation as they battle phantom pain, it tends to improve gradually.

Torticollis

These are muscle spasms to one side of the neck. Torticollis literally means turned neck. These sometimes force the head to turn to the side, or sometimes prevent the neck from turning. It can be unsightly and is quite painful.

Torticollis can be caused by an injury or orthopedic condition which can be corrected surgically. A number of muscle-relaxing drugs can also be helpful.

One patient I had with torticollis was Colleen. Colleen was an executive who traveled a great deal, had a tight schedule and many meetings, and the responsibility for many decisions. She came into the office one day with her head firmly twisted to the side. Her chin was almost resting on her right shoulder. There was a visible strain in her neck muscles.

She had already been to other doctors, who had tried a number of treatments. However, she had not tried one thing—stress reduction. She had not tried to use her mind, nor had she tried to be the most active player on her health care team.

Colleen embarked upon a stress reduction program. She adjusted her work schedule, used Relaxation
Response techniques, and quickly improved. When
she meditated, she concentrated on relaxing her neck
muscles—this relaxation routine worked.

Cancer Pain

Everyone fears cancer. Many people fear the idea
of dying less than the thought of living for weeks or
months with severe pain.

Many cancers do not cause pain in the beginning
stages. Therefore, these types of cancer are often not
diagnosed until the disease has progressed significantly.
However, many cancers cause a great deal of pain,
especially when bones are involved.

The good news is that there are new ways of
giving medications. Some of these ways work quite
well in reducing pain.

1.   Bone pain often responds to anti-inflammatory drugs like aspirin and ibuprofen. They are especially effective when combined with narcotics. In fact,
less narcotics can be used if you combine these nonpre-
scription drugs with anti-inflammatories.

2.   Slow release capsules that have been
recently developed are good ways of treating pain in a
timed, specific fashion. This helps prevent addiction.

3.   Doctors can give pain-relieving drugs

straight into the vein, with a release button; a patient taught to use this technique can give himself a dose if the pain gets severe. Of course, limits are programmed into the machine to prevent overdoses.

4.   Skin patches that release small amounts of narcotics into the skin for twenty-four hours usually have some effectiveness.

5.   Electronic stimuli such as a TENS machine may reduce cancer pain. Some machines can stimulate specific parts of the spinal cord.

A large number of states have changed their laws regarding the use of narcotics. The federal government has yet to follow suit. An important factor to consider in dealing with cancer pain is that it usually can be controlled with proper medication.

Many measures avoid the pitfalls of typical injected medication where the patient wavers between deep sleep and deep pain. Quality of life can be improved or preserved.

Chapter 7

Special Pain Treatments

In your battle against pain, you will discover that certain medical treatments are necessary and helpful. For instance, a properly placed nerve block can make a huge difference in certain cases. Other treatments such as electric stimulation can also help your physical problems.

Beyond the specific physical benefit of a treatment, there is a secondary benefit. A treatment often has symbolic value to a patient. It is important for you to know that your suffering is being taken seriously. A physical treatment makes you more alert and inclined to listen to your doctor's advice.

For a physician, pain is a byproduct of illnesses or accidents. Pain is not the cause of physical problems. Thus, your pain is not the focus of their study of your physical condition. A physician will try and relieve your pain. If the pain persists, your physician may recommend you see a pain specialist at a pain clinic.

At a pain clinic, there are specialists in Anesthesiology, Physical Therapy, Occupational Therapy, Industrial Medicine, Psychology, Psychiatry, Neurology, Neuro Surgery, and Orthopedic Surgery among others.

At a pain clinic, the pain itself is the entire focus of the care team. A pain specialist accepts without hesitation that you have pain. And a pain specialist has an arsenal of measures which can be used to improve your situation.

:60 Second Special Treatments List

1.	Mechanical Adjustments in the Workplace
2.	TENS Machine
3.	Nerve Blocks, Shots
4.	Biofeedback
5.	Exercise
6.	Walking
7.	A Simple, or Elegant Cane
8.	Hot and Cold Applications

Mechanical Adjustments in the Workplace

Once you have accepted the fact that your pain is not imagined, you can begin to deal with it. This means doing what you can to make the pain less debilitating.

The first two places to look for factors to change are your workplace and home. Anything that can be done to make work easier should be done. *Comfort at work is not a luxury*, rather it is a necessity. The same is true for someone doing housework. Work at home involves a lot of standing and bending, which can be painful. You can make a simple adjustment just by purchasing three inexpensive stools. The simple, unpainted kind is fine. A low stool is useful for gardening and working on the floor. A medium stool is good for work at a table. And a high stool (a bar stool) is good for work on a kitchen counter.

If you do desk work, whether at an office or at home, make allowances for the pain you feel and accommodate these problems. In some cases, work is only possible if proper adjustments are made. They make you more productive.

A comfortable chair at work may be your most important tool. The chair should be the proper height for your legs and for your desk. Some adjustments may be necessary in the table height or chair height to diminish strain. A keyboard and monitor should be positioned properly for those who work on a computer. These adjustments are minor, but they are essential for good concentration and performance.

In factory work, placement of machines, handles, and other controls has become a science. Insurance companies are very interested in this factor because it promotes safety as well as efficiency. Proper lighting is also essential for safety and healthy eyesight.

Music during work can have a calming or inspiring

effect on your attitude.

The best way to cope with physical difficulties at work is to adjust the way you work. You can do it if you want to do it. Your mind is stronger than your body, and the workplace is one place where you can illustrate that fact.

TENS Machine

The actual name of this machine used for physical therapy is Transcutaneous Electronic Nerve Stimulator. The word transcutaneous means "through the skin." A TENS machine consists of a control box, wires, and sticky electrodes. The electrodes, which resemble band aids, are placed in certain spots near the nerves that lead to painful areas. These spots are called "trigger points." When touched, the trigger points can cause pain elsewhere.

The stimulator, in effect, promotes the production of endorphins, the narcotic-like substances that help the body fight pain. This happens in an area of the spinal cord, the posterior horn, and where the pain and the touch nerves meet.

The touch nerves are larger and produce stronger electrical signals than the thin pain nerves. The successful reaction of a TENS machine follows the Gate Theory (referred to in Chapter 1). The touch nerves are stimulated, thus overriding the pain felt in the pain nerves.

Frequently, the best policy is to bracket the pain—placing one electrode above the pain and one below the pain. If there are two sets of electrodes, the same is done with the second pair.

When the electrodes have been properly placed, the patient is instructed to turn on the control button very slowly until he or she feels a gentle tingle. This amount of current is often sufficient for good results. Sometimes a stronger current is required. The current should never rise to a level where the muscles start twitching.

When a TENS machine works well, pain begins to ease within a half hour. The machine is kept working for a while and results are observed. The machine should be stopped a few times, for about two-hour stretches; so the body does not grow too habituated to it. It is not advisable to use a TENS machine while you sleep.

People who wear an electronic cardiac pacemaker should not use a TENS machine, because it could interfere with the signal of the pacemaker. Some people with heart and eye conditions should not use the TENS machine either (discuss this with your regular doctor).

TENS machines work for about sixty percent of those who use them properly.

Frank and the TENS Machine

Frank, a retiree in his seventies, has hypertrophic facet joint disease. This disease affects the small joints in the back which make a twisting motion possible. He had significant pain, due to this disease.

Frank had serious pains in his lower back, groin, and knee. He had no trigger points, and tests for disc disease were negative. Still, he had pain, and he attributed much of it to tension.

Frank had had many different treatments, but none were successful until I started him on a TENS machine. It was immediately helpful. He felt better when upright and soon was able to start going to church. Frank also resumed walking. He could even turn the machine off for a few hours at a time so he could swim. That exercise helped him even more.

After Frank had adjusted to the TENS unit, he started Relaxation Response. He learned quickly and practiced regularly. He began to do other physical exercises. This combination of relaxation exercises, a TENS unit, and physical exercise worked out well. Frank's state of mind improved; he began enjoying life more; and his pain diminished markedly.

Nerve Blocks, Shots

In many chronic pain situations, the question of needle treatments will inevitably come up. Nerve blocks can be very helpful and they are safe in experienced hands.

There are two types of nerve blocks:

1.   Diagnostic nerve blocks are used to determine which nerves are involved in the pain problems. Nerves that are suspected of being involved in pain are injected with a local anesthetic solution. If the pain stops after the injection of the block; then the origin of the pain is likely to be in the area of the nerve or nerves that were blocked. If you block the nerves that are presumed to cause the pain and the pain doesn't stop, it means the pain is located either in the spine or a memory center in the brain.

Another form of diagnostic nerve blocks are sympathetic nerve blocks. These cause a relaxation of blood vessels, especially when those vessels are in spasm. These will also cause a warming of the skin in the blocked area. This kind of nerve block, though effective in treating pain (especially sympathetic dystrophy and shingles), can also be used in helping a surgeon decide whether an operation would be useful.

2.   Therapeutic blocks are also used to treat chronic pain. There are many kinds:

Triggerpoint blocks are the injections of anesthetics into trigger points near the area of pain. (As was explained earlier, a trigger point is a spot which, when touched, causes pain elsewhere.) When the injection is composed of an anesthetic mixed with a steroid, it can be very helpful.

Steroid epidural blocks put a steroid near the nerve roots in the epidural space of the spinal cord. The epidural space is an area around the spinal cord and out-side of the sac that holds the spinal fluid. The nerve roots in the epidural space can become thick and swollen from a herniated disk. A steroid can reduce the swelling.

Facet blocks are injections given under x-ray control into one of the small slanted joints (called facet joints) that are between the vertebrae.

Therapeutic infiltration is an injection of a local anesthetic and a steroid into a painful area of shingles. This works, but not on everyone.

Intravenous Xylocaine treatment is an intra-venous drip solution. A needle is inserted into a vein, and a solution such as normal saline is mixed with a local anesthetic called Xylocaine. The solution stabilizes membranes, often nerve fibers. This can be especially beneficial in certain cases of diabetes by reducing the activity in painful nerves. The patient must be lying or sitting down as the treatment can make him/her quite dizzy.

Permanent blocks will not necessarily last forever. Attempts can be made to block nerves with alcohol or phenol to stop the activity in those nerves. This is done with great caution so as to be sure not to inject unin-volved nerves. The problem is that those nerves can recover in three months, and yet, the pain can end up much worse. Therefore, this procedure is used with extreme care and only administered in special cases, such as to patients with severe cancers.

Biofeedback

Not everyone needs biofeedback. Many people can learn Relaxation Response exercises quite well. Many also become adept at visual imagery. (These are methods that were discussed in Chapter 4).

However, some people need help learning to control those body responses which are not normally under conscious control. Biofeedback is a process which measures many bodily responses and displays them to a patient in ways that are easy to understand. The responses that can be measured include:

1.   Muscle tension and relaxation
2.   Skin temperature
3.   Brain waves

By watching the machine, an experienced patient can learn to control those responses.

:60 Second Biofeedback Information

1.   The amount of electric currents (action currents) that occur before or during muscle contraction are measured by the biofeedback machine. A completely relaxed muscle will display little or no reading on the dial, but a muscle in contraction or spasm will display a higher reading. Electrodes are placed around the muscle group to be relaxed, and the patient learns to watch the

dial for reactions. Some machines make sounds to make observations easier. The idea behind this is for the patient to learn the procedure so well that they can produce relaxation without the aid of the machine.

2.   Heat sensing electrodes are applied to the skin to measure skin temperature. When no specific areas are indicated, this may be on the skin of the forehead or arm. If the patient gets into a relaxed (meditative) state, the skin temperature tends to rise slightly. The reactions are displayed on a dial, which the patient should learn so well as to be able to learn to relax without the machine.

Sometimes the aim is to improve circulation in a specific area of the body. In that case, heat sensitive electrodes are placed on the skin of the area to be treated. The patient then tries relaxation or visual imagery, and can see on the dial whether it is working.

3.   Electrodes are placed on the scalp and the machine displays brain waves. Again, the patient is taught techniques to reach a relaxed or meditative state, and can watch the dial to see progress.

However, there are drawbacks. This is an expensive treatment method and it does not work for many people experiencing chronic pain.

It has worked well for some with tension headaches, migraines, TMJ disease, and several other conditions. It may work for you.

:60 Second Exercise Information

1.	Exercise leads to physical improvement.
2.	Exercise leads to improvement in mood and self esteem.
3.	It may hurt a little, but it won't hurt you.
4.	Pace yourself, don't race.

:60 Second Simple Exercise Chart

1.	Walking
2.	Swimming
3.	Water gymnastics
4.	Waterwalking
5.	Stretching exercises
6.	Floor gymnastics
7.	Aerobics
8.	Nautilus and similar equipment
9.	Stationary or regular bicycles

1.   Walking can be one of the happiest experiences of a lifetime. Immediate rewards as well as long-term benefits can be the results of walking. For example, walking offers tranquility. It also gives you a good opportunity to do some relaxed thinking, meditating, or daydreaming. Walking provides many more physical and psychic benefits.

Still, it can be difficult to start the habit of walking if you are used to a sedentary lifestyle. It is even more difficult for someone whose pain interferes with the act of walking. But if you start slowly, you can succeed.

Begin with a five-minute walk and gradually work your way up to longer ones. Whenever possible, walk in a scenic area where you can see some trees, bushes, flowers, and people. Parks often make very good walking sites.

In bad weather, you can walk in a mall. "Mall hopping" is a favorite activity of many people. There are often benches in malls, which is helpful for someone trying to build a new walking routine.

Some like the solitude of a walk alone, while others prefer walking in company. Whatever the case, both have benefits, mental and physical to offer.

2.   Swimming is one of the best exercises for limbering up one's body. Use whatever swimming method suits you, and build up your program gradually.

Start with a few laps of freestyle, breast stroke, back stroke, side stroke, or whatever stroke you can perform with relative ease. A slight ache in the muscles is a useful warning sign that it may be time for a rest. Take a little rest and then go back in the water. Increase your efforts gradually.

3.   Water gymnastics is ideal for many people in chronic pain. You weigh a great deal less in the water,

and it is easier to move stiff muscles. The pain that can be caused by weight is reduced greatly, yet you still receive beneficial exercise. Inform the instructor about any limitations you may have, including your doctor's suggestions regarding pulse rate.

4.   Waterwalking is also ideal. In the water, you can take big steps, raise your legs, walk backwards, walk sideways to your left and then to your right. This freedom is yours.

5.   Stretching exercises are wonderful, especially for people with lower back problems, but they must be designed for you by a physiotherapist or an instructor.

6.   Floor gymnastics have a distinct advantage in that they can be done at home. Remember, a slight ache is a healthy ache.

7.   Aerobics are designed to raise your pulse rate and oxygen consumption. Low impact aerobics can be very beneficial, but may be too strenuous for some individuals. Be sure to check with your doctor before starting aerobics.

8.   Nautilus and similar equipment may do a great deal to strengthen your back and your muscles. Get advice from an instructor or physiotherapist before

starting to use this equipment.

9.   Stationary or regular bicycles work your muscles and your cardiovascular system. If you have used your bicycle fairly regularly in the past, it is a good idea to take it up again. But if you haven't used one in years, I would not encourage the experiment. A stationary bicycle is less risky and very convenient. You can listen to a radio or watch television to reduce boredom.

:60 Second Exercise Summary

---

1.   The fact that you climbed Mount Everest thirty years ago should have no influence on your present program. Do what you can do in light of your physical condition. Don't push to do what you used to do.
2.   Exercising in groups is preferable, especially in a noncompetitive setting.
3.   No matter how you exercise, do it regularly—at least five times a week.

A Simple or Fancy Cane

Canes are on the borderline between medical supports and fancy accessories. In past centuries, a cane was a fashion statement.

Anyone who uses a cane should not feel that it makes them look impaired or handicapped. Quite the contrary. A cane shows that you want to walk, and that you want to walk further.

Canes are useful, are not addicting, and do not cause dependency. Simply put, if used properly, a cane can aid your walking ability and endurance. When a cane is used correctly, it reduces weight that hips, knees, and lower back support.

A cane is normally placed in the hand away from your pain. If both sides are painful, you will have to develop a system of changing hands every fifty or so steps. This way you can aid both areas.

A cane must be the proper length. I recommend it have a bent crook so you can hang it over your arm when you are at rest.

Unless, for some reason, your doctor recommends a metal cane, I recommend a wooden one. It does not proclaim you as a sick or handicapped person, and therefore that label does not impinge on your conscious mind. If you pick out an elegant wooden cane, light and sturdy, you can make it part of your personality. The message is clear: I want to walk.

Hot and Cold Applications

There are some simple and inexpensive ways to relieve pain. Hot and cold applications fall into this category.

The question is, which is better? Hot or cold? There is not a simple answer. Individuals respond differently. You have to try both methods yourself.

:60 Second System for Hot and Cold Applications

1.   Test your own responses by trying hot and cold applications at different times.
2.   For spastic muscles, I recommend hot applications.
3.   When nerves are irritated, as in neuralgia, neuritis, or neuropathy, I suggest an application of cold water or an ice bag. I have found these to be most effective.
4.   Many muscle or nerve pains respond well to the freeze and move method.

:60 Second Methods for Applying Heat or Cold

1.   Heat is best applied with a hot water bottle or a heating pad. Please note, do not use these devices while asleep or when numbness is present. There is a possibility of burns.
2.   Cold can be applied by applying an ice bag or positioning an aching body part under an ice cold water tap.
3.   The freeze and move method is particularly effective for many pain situations. You apply ice to a painful area for about ten minutes or until numb, then move the area gently. This is particularly effective for sprains, bursitis, tendinitis, and other conditions.

Ted's Story

Ted came to my office to discuss a work injury to his foot and lower leg. A heavy object had fallen on him. Afterward, he began experiencing pain down the lower left side of both his legs, and from his left lower back down to his left big toe. His left foot tended to get numb.

He had had an operation on his back and two steroid epidural blocks, but there was no significant improvement in the pain he was experiencing.

When I first saw Ted, he weighed 240 pounds. He drank several six packs of beer every week, smoked one pack of cigarettes a day, and had, at least, four servings of caffeine daily (coffee and cola).

I talked to him about his faulty diet, smoking, consumption of alcohol, and intake of caffeine. During the week which followed, he quit drinking, cut down on caffeine, and started losing weight. His attitude improved and he began exercising.

I tried using a trigger point block at this point, and Ted received relief for almost two weeks. Next, I tried using spinal facet blocks, which gave him relief for four months. These blocks were given in the small joints on the vertebrae (facets) that make twisting and bending possible. When Ted felt better, he adopted a more rigorous exercise program, which relieved his chronic pain even more.

The crucial message is that Ted changed his lifestyle. Once he understood and acted on his destructive behavior patterns, the medical techniques we used on his pain worked.

Chapter 8

Medications

Do not believe that the medications you are taking will make your pain disappear forever. If you have such expectations, you have missed the point of this book and possibly set yourself up for crushing disappointment.

Remember that medications are not 100 percent successful. Moreover, they only work for a limited time.

A better approach to using medications is to expect that they help in dealing with your pain for a period. Understand that medication may not eliminate *all* of your pain. Accept that medication is a tool to help you function more efficiently and happily.

With chronic pain, you should look for step-by-step improvement, not a cure. Remember to pace yourself, and don't expect miracles.

:60 Second Medication Rules

1.   Take your medicine *exactly as ordered*. If it is intended for severe pain only, don't take it at regular intervals in the absence of pain. If, however, it is intended to be taken at regular intervals, don't reserve it for severe pain only.

2.   Most drugstores furnish you with warnings of possible side reactions and complications. Pay close attention to this advice.

3.   Follow the instructions. If you are supposed to take your medication after meals, don't take it on an empty stomach.

4.   Don't increase or decrease dosage without permission.

5.   Report side effects to your doctor at once.

6.   Be patient. Many medications do not work at once. The substance must build up in your blood. This can take days or even weeks.

7.   Be careful not to stop certain medications suddenly. You can experience unpleasant side effects.

8.   All effective medications are bound to produce some side reactions. Be alert to them.

9.   Do not rely on medication alone.

Willpower and Pill Power

If you follow your doctor's directions on medications exactly, you should not run into any complications.

However, if you take medications on your own or if you stop medications without advice from your doctor, you can get into major trouble.

For people with certain conditions or illnesses, some prescribed medications are essential for life and functioning. They cannot be stopped in the foreseeable future without serious complications. Other medications can be stopped, but only gradually to avoid unpleasant reactions such as withdrawal. If you wean the body from a drug, the body is better able to handle the change. Of course, your mind still has a great deal of control.

Consider the case of Robert, who had severe shooting pain in his legs from neuritis, an inflammation of the nerve. In addition to pain, he felt numbness. His neuritis probably was caused by his diabetes.

When Robert first visited, I put him on regular doses of Dilantin. I expected success because this treatment usually works in such cases. But Robert returned and said he was not better.

I ordered a blood test on Robert. When the test revealed he had almost no Dilantin in his blood, I knew there was a problem. If he had taken regular doses as instructed, his blood level would have contained the amount of medicine required to be effective.

It turned out that Robert had decided to take the

Dilantin only when he felt intolerable pain. He skipped daily doses.

"I thought it would do more good," he said.

Different medications work different ways, and your doctor knows just how it should be administered to alleviate your problem. Changing a medication schedule on your own is unwise, and it can be dangerous. Listen to your doctor.

Anti-Inflammatory Drugs

Anti-inflammatories reduce inflammation. There are two categories of these drugs:

1.   Steroids
2.   Non-steroids

1.   Steroids are hormones originally derived from the adrenal gland. Many of them can now be produced synthetically. Prednisone, Cortisone, and other types of steroids are particularly helpful in treating certain forms of arthritis, such as rheumatoid arthritis. Steroids also reduce allergic reactions, some diseases, and some severe cases of asthma.

Although, steroids can be useful, there are also a long list of side reactions which may occur, including: salt retention, water retention, and increased blood pressure and pulse rate. Some patients develop ulcers, while others experience mood changes or even mental disturbances. If taken for a long period of time, steroids interfere with the immune system.

Certainly, the risks may make you wonder why take steroids at all. The answer is that your physician carefully weighs the benefit and risk relationship. In some cases, the benefits outweigh the risks.

2. Non-steroid anti-inflammatory drugs, such as aspirin, have great usefulness for those who can take them. Within limits, they are good temporary pain relievers. They also reduce fever and are of particular value in the battle against bone cancer pain. They actually lessen the amount of narcotics needed to keep this kind of severe pain in check.

These drugs also have potential problems, such as producing ulcers and increased bleeding, especially for those with a sensitive gastrointestinal system. The function of blood clotting can be disturbed as well.

Millions take these drugs without complication, while others taking them have problems. Therefore, be aware and ask your doctor for instructions.

Acetaminophen

The common brand name of this drug is Tylenol. It can be used to reduce fevers, as it tends to dull the pain sensation.

Acetaminophen is not an anti-inflammatory medicine, nor is it expected to have a great effect on arthritis or similar complaints. However, it does not cause the same afflictions, such as stomach problems and increased threat of bleeding, that anti-inflammatories do. Instead, you run the risk of liver or kidney damage if overdosed or taken for too long.

The discovery that this "harmless" drug has side effects was quite a disappointment, but keep in mind that any effective medicine is bound to have side reactions.

One final note: people who consume alcohol and take Tylenol are more prone to major side reactions.

Anti-Convulsant Drugs

These drugs slow down certain chemical reactions that cause or are caused by hyperexcitability. Anti-convulsant drugs work especially well on epilepsy. Phenytoin and carbamazepine are the most common anti-convulsant drugs. However, both Dilantin, a form of phenytoin, and Tegretol, a form of carbamazepine, have benefits that need to be seriously weighed against their many side effects.

Dilantin is especially useful for people who feel lightning-like attacks of pain. However, it is only effective when there is a certain level of the drug in the bloodstream. Regular doses are necessary.

The dosage should be watched closely because of Dilantin's side effects. When an overdose occurs, it can interfere with the production of vitamin D (which benefits the bones). Dilantin can also interfere with the release of insulin, causing blood sugar to become higher than normal. Confusion, skin rashes, or swollen gums can occur as side effects as well.

Alcohol should not be consumed in conjunction with this drug, because it can cause excessive sleepiness. Dilantin is metabolized in the liver; a potential problem for some liver patients.

Most people can take Dilantin safely, but every patient should watch for warning signs.

Tegretol is very effective, almost remarkable, in treating a type of severe pain in the face called trigeminal neuralgia.

However, the drug has an even longer list of side effects than Dilantin. It may cause damage to bone marrow or interfere with the production of blood cells. It can also cause severe anemia or a catastrophic lack of immune cells.

There may be symptoms such as dizziness, confusion, or other neurological or psychiatric changes. People with glaucoma may experience increased pressure in the eye. There can be skin rashes, elevated blood pressure, and heart problems as well.

This does not mean the drug is useless. It simply means that precautions must be taken when this drug is ordered for a patient. These precautions include periodic blood counts and frequent reporting by the individual, so that the first signs of a complication are noted and acted upon.

Narcotics

Although narcotics are discussed in the chapter on habits, it is important to understand the medical thinking behind the use or non-use of narcotic medications.

There are several classes of drugs involved which have a variety of uses.

1.   Mild narcotics such as Codeine, Percocet, and mixtures containing these substances and other drugs are useful in alleviating acute pain; especially when there is no longer the need for injected medication. These milder pain relievers are helpful in postoperative pain as well.

There is little or no argument regarding the use of narcotics when a patient is experiencing acute pain, although care still must be taken to avoid side reactions.

However, use of them in cases of chronic pain is not the preference of some doctors. Others say the judicious use of moderate doses can assure some patients will be able to have useful lives.

The problem is that there is no way of identifying which patients will not develop an addiction. Each patient's history must be evaluated. If the patient has any history of addiction (to alcohol or any medicine), it is advisable not to use narcotics with that individual.

2.   Strong narcotics include medicines such as Demerol or Morphine and are usually injected under

the skin or into a muscle. The best method of administering these drugs is the injection of small doses repeated at frequent intervals. Sometimes, patients can be hooked up to a machine that allows them to push a button to give themselves effective doses. This machine has a security lock to prevent patients from taking overdoses.

3.   Strong narcotics prescribed in a long-lasting form are especially useful in the home treatment of cancer pain. The narcotic is given in slow-release form so that two or three doses a day may be enough.

4.   Short-acting narcotics such as Fentanyl can be injected or used in the form of a skin patch. This is especially useful in postoperative pain.

5.   Narcotic antagonists counteract the effect of a narcotic immediately. These agents have saved many lives in cases of overdose, but are so effective that they can also induce acute withdrawal syndrome.

6.   Agonist-antagonist mixtures such as Talwin are combinations of an active drug and a counter agent in the hope of avoiding complications, especially respiratory depression.

7.   Long-lasting narcotics such as Methadone have been used to wean people from addiction without

major withdrawal symptoms.

All of these drugs can be wonderfully effective with some pain problems, but they must be treated with respect and careful attention.

Medications Applied Externally

People who have aches and pains often apply ointments and creams to aching parts of their bodies. Some "rubs" create a feeling of heat that can be quite soothing. Others, like mineral ice, feel very cool.

Some athletic rubs work on the principle of counter irritation by producing strong feelings short of outright pain on the skin, and help sufferers to overlook their original pains. The explanation for these may lie in the Gate Theory. (See Chapter 1.)

In the last few years, pepper extract creams from Jalapeno peppers have been used to alleviate pain. When applied, these ointments or creams cause feelings of warmth, like sunburn, which frequently reduces pain.

:60 Second Medication Summary

---
1. Medications can be of great help if properly used. But remember that most of your pain control depends on you.
2. You cannot control your pain if you cannot control your intake of medicines.
3. Don't depend on medicines. Depend on yourself. Remember that your mind is stronger than your body.

Chapter 9

Keeping Track

You may believe your condition will improve or perhaps just hope that it will happen. In either case, you must realize that improvement will be a slow and gradual process.

If you don't keep track, you may miss the first signs of improvement. It is essential to mark your progress in a number of areas including: pain level, mood, smoking, medications, alcohol, calories, weight, and activities. Do this every day, and you will have a record to which you can refer to showing your progress.

The chart which follows is useful in keeping track of many aspects of pain management.

Fill in the chart on the next page.

:60 SECOND PAIN MANAGEMENT CHART

Time	Mood 0-10	Pain 0-10	Medication, Dosage Time	TENS +/-	Activities Letter Code	Remarks Location of Pain
8 A.M.						
9 A.M.						
10 A.M.						
11 A.M.						
12 Noon						
1 P.M.						
2 P.M.						
3 P.M.						
4 P.M.						
5 P.M.						
6 P.M.						
7 P.M.						
8 P.M.						
9 P.M.						
10 P.M.						
11 P.M.						
12 Mid to 8 A.M.						

:60 Second Pain Management
Chart Instructions

Mood Score:
0   = You feel alert, active, awake, and happy.
1-5 = Closer to happy.
6-9 = Closer to sad.
10 = You feel sad, depressed, useless, nearly desperate.

Pain Score:
0   = No pain at all.
1-2 = Slight pain that does not interfere with life.
3-5 = Quite disagreeable pain.
6-7 = So painful you must stop activities.
8-9 = Very painful and distressing.
10 = The worst pain imaginable.

Medications With Dosage And Time:
 The idea is to see how medications relate to pain level. Include all medications (from over-the-counter to external ones), alcohol, and caffeine on your chart.

TENS:
 When the machine is on, mark a "+" and when it is off, mark a "-".

Activities:

Here is a letter code to avoid a lot of writing. If you do something different, use your own abbreviations.

A.   Eating
B.   Sleeping
C.   Resting
D.   Watching television
E.   Walking
F.   Working
G.   Exercising
H.   Gardening
I.   Hobbies (music, painting, woodworking, etc.)
J.   Reading
K.   Driving
L.   Traveling
M.   Education (taking courses, home study, etc.)
N.   Working around the home
O.   Yard work
P.   Cooking

Chapter 10

Final Briefing,
The Future

Chronic pain does not have to shut down your active life. In fact, chronic pain presents you with an opportunity for a better life if you look at it as a choice. If you have ruled out suffering constantly, then there is really only one option—control.

This means changing your life. When you have chronic pain, you lead a life in which there are some limitations. But there are also new options. Options of the mind. By challenging yourself in new ways, you can find new strengths. These can be very different from those you possessed in your old life. However, your mind has incredible powers to adapt, and to override.

One sad part about chronic pain is that some things can't be taken for granted anymore. See these as new challenges.

I did not write this book to tell you that your pain will disappear. I am a doctor, not a magician. The message of this book is that for improvement to occur, you must be involved in your care, not just a bystander. This book also gives a message from my heart saying I understand, and here are some ideas and treatments that I have seen help.

Control

As a word, "control" means manage, govern, rule. As a philosophy, it means discipline, restraint, courage, and action. When you control something, you don't expect it to vanish completely.

If, for example, you try to control a river, you don't expect to eliminate the river. You establish boundaries for its everyday flow, and also emergency boundaries so that it can overflow without doing damage.

Likewise, if you control the temperature in your house, you do not eliminate all temperature. You just eliminate the extremes of hot and cold.

With pain control, you also eliminate the extremes. All pain may not be gone, but it is diminished. And you want to be able to do this without losing all feeling and becoming numb.

Control is not an easy task although it is a simple concept. You can control, within limits, your walking speed. You can control, within limits, the clothes you wear.

And you can control your reaction to pain.

But to establish control, you must first experience the feeling of *being in control*. There are specific tools involved. Conscious decisions. Start with a small task just to prove how a conscious decision works. For example, right now I want you to decide to take a breath. See. You can exercise self control. You can make this process grow so that certain things that are not necessarily as effortless as taking a breath can be controlled by you.

You can also decide not to do some things that are not good for you.

Increase your self control. *Your mind is stronger than your body.* Whether you decide to take a breath, or do something much more difficult, you have the power to improve your life. When you get control, you get a special feeling. A feeling of power, even over small matters.

In this book, you have learned many ways to gain control of chronic pain. You have learned about medications, outside stimulation, relaxation response, visualization, and override. These are treatments and techniques. If pain relieving treatments are prescribed, take them. As for techniques, learn them.

Control requires constant effort. It is not easy, but the effect on your life and pain is more than worth it.

:60 Second Steps Toward Pain Control

1.	Follow your doctor's orders
2.	Stay positive
3.	Practice relaxation and visualization
4.	Be careful of habits
5.	Stay active and exercise
6.	Keep track of improvements
7.	Do things for others
8.	Rest when necessary
9.	Believe in something
10.	Believe in yourself

Start Planning Your New Life

Think of a list—things to do to improve your life and diminish your pain. Start with ideas for improvements. Say, "When I have less pain, I will do this . . ." List positive things. Don't daydream about the impossible. Write down still do-able objectives or things you want to or can almost do.

What pleasurable tasks and events do you want to perform? And, if you are already doing them, could you do them better, with more cheer. Could you smile, even if it takes some effort?

Don't even think about tackling every item on your list at once. Don't set yourself up for failure. Set yourself up for success.

The Actual List

Start with a small one--three items. From there, narrow it to one. Try it.

Go for that walk. Make it to religious services. Visit your friends. Go shopping. Smile around your family. Make the effort. Trying will make you feel good about yourself.

The best part is if you make a realistic list, you will succeed. Then you will get more control and more confidence. And when your mind is confident, it can do amazing things.

Do Things

Life is an adventure, an open road, but as you travel this road, you are bound to hit a few bumps. When this happens to someone with chronic pain, it is easy to think the road comes to a stop. However, the road goes on. There are new experiences waiting for you, and even when you are experiencing chronic pain, you can enjoy the bounty of life.

Cultivate the habit of being active. This is a big step to getting back into life.

Many chronic pain sufferers tend to be afraid of being active for fear of hurting themselves further. This inertia is self defeating. It leads to more pain because muscles become rigid. That is physical pain. The real pain, though, is more than physical. It is both emotional and mental. The mind as well as the body becomes rigid and stiff. It's a trap.

The best way to break out of the trap is to start doing small things. Don't worry about the big things. You can tackle them in the course of time. The important step is making a beginning, getting started.

PRO-Gram and ANTI-Gram

Plan your activities so that the things you attempt can be accomplished with some degree of satisfaction and without too much discomfort. Call this your PRO-Gram.

Also, keep in mind that some of your activities may cause you pain. That is called your ANTI-Gram. Your ANTI-Gram is against you.

PRO-Gram literally translated means something written beforehand. Your PRO-Gram should be a plan for your benefit.

Build your "PRO" plan around achievable results, so that each accomplishment will cause good and happy feelings.

An ANTI-Gram is a plan that cannot be carried out without negative consequences. If you decide to shovel snow and declare you'll clear the whole side-walk, you may be setting yourself up for failure as well as pain. If you feel you must rake the whole lawn now, you may be setting yourself up for an impossible task—an ANTI-gram. Although your intentions in such a case may be good, the logic is faulty.

In your new life plan, set yourself up for success. Don't set unreasonable goals. Know what your limits are and adapt. Plan rest periods—frequent and short activity is better than constant and long activity.

Plan your day. Plan for something good to happen every day. It can be a little goal, such as a short stroll, going on an automobile ride, reading a book, or watching a favorite television show. Of course, if your choice is watching a television show, make it a special one. Don't spend all day in front of the tube. Call on a friend. Perhaps you can't do this every day, but make the effort to do it more frequently.

Remember, anything that can brighten your day will make your pain a little less difficult to bear, so plan for these activities.

Know Your Limitations

To set yourself up for success, you must know your limitations. To know them, you have to test them from time to time.

:60 Second Limitations Guide

> •If you can walk five minutes, try six.
> •If you can swim one length of the pool, try two.
> •If you can sit up and read for thirty minutes,
> try thirty-five.
> •If you can perform an exercise twice, try to do it
> three times.
> •If you spend four hours out of twenty-four on your
> feet and you spend twenty lying down, try five up
> and nineteen down.

If you succeed and make progress, test your new limit.

If you fail, don't be discouraged. Recognize your limit and work with it. Remember to test it again in the future.

When you succeed, rejoice in your success. Mark it in your diary. Mark it in your mental diary as well. Give yourself a gold star. Congratulate yourself. Don't let success, no matter how small, go unnoticed. Instead, build from it.

Limit Your Limitation

Think of a limitation as a challenge. Train your mind to think positive thoughts. Don't think unrealistic thoughts. Don't pretend that you can change a limitation overnight. It may take a while. But start to push the edges a little.

Know your limitations, and then limit your limitations.

Priorities

If you decide that pain is the most important thing in your life, pain and suffering will dominate your life experience. This will have a major influence on your attitude and your pain experience.

You are the only person on earth who is able to decide your priorities. You do it consciously and unconsciously.

For instance, imagine you are to meet an old and good friend whom you have not seen in a long while. This event is the most important thing on your mind. It conjures up emotions, memories, and expectations. Your pain takes a back seat. The pain does not vanish, but your mental reaction to it is postponed, at least until the friendly reunion is over. When you do this, you are postponing the mental reaction to pain.

Suffering is a mental reaction to pain, it is the most difficult part of the pain experience. And so, to avoid suffering by postponing pain is to lessen the pain experience.

The question is, "After a few hours of postponing pain, what do you do next?"

Find something else to take the priority spot.

Put this thing first. It works.

For instance, I worked for quite a few years while enduring hip arthritis that was very painful, but my work was so interesting that I didn't notice the pain while I was trying to help my patients. Of course, not everybody has an interesting and exciting job. But you can still succeed in postponing the pain experience.

Make a list of activities to push ahead of pain. Don't make the list too long. If it fits on a three-inch by five-inch file card, keep the card with you at all times. Underline the items that work best. Use those most frequently. Prioritize. Remember that your mind is stronger than your body. Don't let your mind be used by your pain.

Instead remember to: *use your mind to diminish suffering. It has enormous power.*

:60 Second Chronic Pain Truths

I have studied pain and its treatment for decades. I have learned a lot, and I tried to share my knowledge with you. My hopes and prayers are with you.

I believe in you. If you have taken control of your life, you believe in yourself too. If you believe in yourself, you will succeed.

In studying my patient's records for this book, I have not only presented the treatments which worked best, but the attitudes which helped most of my patients get better.

:60 Second Summary

1. They wanted to get better.
2. They believed their efforts would bring about desired results.
3. They accepted the fact that their pain existed and were ready to cope with it.
4. They noted and rejoiced in every small success or improvement.
5. They noted setbacks only for the purpose of learning from them.
6. They learned that a person suffering chronic pain must have patience and not expect huge changes in one day.
7. They found out that success is bought with sacrifice. They learned to do things of benefit, such as exercise, and to give up cherished bad habits, like smoking.
8. They decided they were the most important member of their health care team and accepted that responsibility while cooperating with the rest of their team.

Postscript

You have embarked upon a journey from pain beyond life, to life beyond pain. Don't deny your pain but rather deny the dominant role it has earlier played. You can be the master of your fate. You can restore the quality of your life.

You can win. You will win.

I know it. You must believe it.

It may take time. Pace yourself. Use the :60 second techniques suggested in this book.

And, as Winston Churchill said, "Never give up. Never, never give up."